JUST DO IT!

Total sexual fitness is finally within your grasp!

Want to rev up your sex drive and boost desire? Try eating cruciferous vegetables like broccoli and cabbage, and add soy products to your diet.

Struggling with impotence? Look to your spice rack for some surprisingly simple answers. Cinnamon, ginseng, or saw palmetto just might do the trick.

Do you long for greater sexual pleasure and enhanced orgasms? Learn the amazing secrets of Kegel exercises. Plus, discover some great couple workouts!

Want to build sexual strength and stamina . . . and reduce stress at the same time? Try qigong, a Chinese discipline that brings together the mind, body, and spirit.

Looking for new ways to awaken your partner's sexual energy? Learn how to perform a sensual massage that transfers energy from one person to another *and* provides physical, emotional, and spiritual revitalization.

Research about sexual health is ongoing and subject to interpretation, and there is no guarantee that what we know about the complex subject won't change with time. The reader should bear in mind that this book is not intended to take the place of medical or psychological advice from a trained professional. Readers are advised to consult a physician or other qualified health professional regarding treatment of all problems relating to sexual health and sexual functioning.

Neither the publisher, the producer, nor the author take any responsibility for any possible consequences from any treatment, action, or application of medicine or preparation to any person reading or following the information in this book.

SEXUAL VIGOR FOR LIFE THE NATURAL WAY

A GUIDE TO TOTAL SEXUAL FITNESS

DEBORAH MITCHELL

Foreword by Sherry Sedgwick, M. Ed.

ibooks
new york
www.ibooks.net

DISTRIBUTED BY PUBLISHERS GROUP WEST

A Publication of ibooks, inc.

Originally published as
Peak Performance: A Guide to Total Sexual Fitness

An ibooks, inc. Book

Distributed by Publishers Group West
1700 Fourth Street, Berkeley, CA 94710
www.pgw.com

ibooks, inc.
24 West 25th Street
New York, NY 10010

The ibooks World Wide Web Site Address is:
www.ibooks.net

ISBN 1-59687-125-3
First ibooks, inc. printing September 2005
10 9 8 7 6 5 4 3 2 1

Interior design by Kate Nichols
Illustrations by Jackie Aher

Printed in the U.S.A.

CONTENTS

FOREWORD

Americans love to think about, and talk about, sex. As a certified sex therapist for more than 15 years, I have heard the stories, fears, joys, and concerns about sex and sexual relationships from thousands of men and women. Regardless of their situations—whether they are single or married; heterosexual, homosexual, or bisexual; regardless of their economic status, age, ethnicity, or race—one basic concept holds true for them and for all sexual adults: Good health is an essential part of healthful, satisfying sex.

Most men and women say they want a fulfilling, healthful sexual relationship, yet many cannot say exactly how to achieve it. They may have heard, for example, that there are ways to strengthen or tone muscles that are used during lovemaking or that can improve the intensity of orgasm, but what are those exercises and how are they done? Perhaps they've wondered about the legendary sexual activities associated with some Eastern cultures but not known where to look for information about those practices. They may know that eating right can help enhance their sex drive, but which foods and supplements in particular are best or "right"? And with all the talk in the media about herbs and the claims that certain ones boost the libido (sexual energy), how do they know which ones really work or how to take those that do work?

Peak Performance: A Guide to Total Sexual Fitness answers these and other questions for anyone who wants to make and keep their sexual relationship healthful and exciting, without the use of drugs or artificial substances. This book has a little something for anyone interested in enhancing his or her sexual relationship. Peak Performance begins with basic information about the functions of the male and female sexual organs and what can happen when something goes awry. These explanations are a good refresher for men and women who think they know what's what but who may have forgotten. Couples who understand the physical factors involved in problems such as impotence and painful intercourse, for example, can be more loving and caring with their partner.

The chapters on foods, supplements, herbs, and homeopathic remedies offer some interesting and easy options couples can use to spice up their sex life and enhance sexual energy. The suggestions are clear and helpful, offering information on how to use the food or remedy and the results you can expect.

For those who hate exercise, the chapter on sexual fitness offers a few twists on tradition: exercises specifically for toning and strengthening sexual muscles, and a series of easy "sexercises" for couples. The sexercises show how sexual fitness can be fun, healthy, and sexy all at the same time, when you share exercise with your sexual partner. And if you ever wanted to explore the sensual world of Eastern sexual methods, this book explains some simple practices you can do right now to promote sexual health and vitality and improve sexual pleasure. The importance of the mind-body connection in sexual health is explored as well, with emphasis on practical methods that are easy to try at home: qigong, yoga, sensate focus exercises, and massage.

This book can be fun and informative for couples who want to enhance their sexual relationship in a natural, healthful way. Put this book on your nightstand or on your coffee table. Share it with your partner. You just might find the peak sexual fitness you've been missing, and thoroughly enjoy the road you take to get there.

Sherry Sedgwick, M.Ed.

CHAPTER ONE

So You Want Great Sex . . .

Sex is on the minds of many people. According to *Sex in America: A Definitive Survey,* results of a sex survey conducted by Edward O. Laumann and fellow researchers at the University of Chicago of more than 3,400 adults show that 54 percent of men think about sex every day or several times a day; another 43 percent think about it a few times a month or a few times a week. Comparable numbers for women are 19 percent and 67 percent. People think about and have sex primarily because it feels good, because they care about or love their partner, and because they want to have children. Whatever the reason, it is natural to want the experience to be as intensely pleasurable as possible. One way to help ensure sexual satisfaction is to be sexually fit and healthy.

For our purposes, sexual fitness means being physically able to participate in sexual activity comfortably and pleasurably, regardless of the form that takes for you; and to attain and maintain a healthy reproductive system to help ensure that sexual encounters are as satisfying as possible and, if desired, that they result in conception. Sexual fitness also involves a degree of emotional and psychological wellness or "fitness." You may be physically capable of engaging in various sexual acts, but that does not mean you are emotionally willing or able to do so. Although this book focuses primarily on physiological fitness for sex, suggestions on how to deal with psychological issues are also provided.

To be sexually fit, there are two areas to consider: overall good health, including proper nutrition, routine exercise, adequate sleep, and other positive lifestyle choices; and situations that present a challenge to sexual activity, such as impotence, menopause, and heart conditions, and natural, safe ways to correct them or make them a positive part of your sexuality. This book helps you achieve sexual fitness and health in both areas. It offers you natural, safe ways to achieve and maintain overall good health and describes holistic approaches to treating conditions that may hinder sexual fitness.

Although this book does *not* teach sexual techniques, it does suggest ways to achieve and maintain optimal physical and mind-body sexual fitness through nutrition and supplementation, herbal medicine, homeopathy, special exercises designed for couples and individuals, and Eastern sexual practices. It is for everyone and anyone who wants to enhance their sexual relationship, improve their fitness level, and become more familiar with how their body and that of their partner can give them pleasure and satisfaction. Whether you or your partner has a sexual problem such as impotence or loss of sexual desire; or a medical condition such as diabetes or heart disease; or simply want to improve your sexual relationship, this book can show you the natural remedies and formulas, the exercises and mind-body experiences, and the foods and supplements that can help you achieve that goal.

Let's begin, however, with a look at sex in America—how much pleasure men and women are getting from their sexual experiences and what types of sexual problems they are having—so you can see where you fit into the country's sexual scene.

Sex in America

You may have heard the expression "If it feels good, do it" ("as long as no one else is hurt in the process"). In days gone by, however, American society viewed sex primarily as a means of procreation and as something men enjoyed but "good girls" didn't. On top of that, sex was rarely discussed, which left many men and women in the dark about what was normal sexual behavior and feelings.

Along came Alfred Charles Kinsey, a sexologist who conducted the first large-scale study of sexual behavior. Kinsey interviewed more than 11,000 men for his study, and in his 1948 book, *Sexual Behavior in the Human Male,* he reported that most men masturbated, most had had premarital sex, and 40 percent of married men had had an extramarital affair. Although his study was criticized for the way the data were obtained, it was groundbreaking in that it burst the puritan view of sex in America. It appeared that people—at least men—were enjoying sex. His 1953 report, *Sexual Behavior in the Human Female,* revealed that women are as capable as men of enjoying sex.

The door to the sexual revolution had begun to open. Kinsey's studies were followed by many others, including those by William H. Masters and Virginia E. Johnson, Shere Hite, Edward Laumann, Cynthia and Samuel Janus, among others. Some of the latest findings show that the men and women who are least satisfied with their sex lives are those who are single, not living with anyone, and who have at least two sexual partners. Only 54 percent of them say they are happy with the physical part of their sexual relationship, and a mere 33 percent are pleased with the emotional side. Among married people, however, up to 88 percent say they are very pleased with the physical portion of their sex lives, while as many as 85 percent say they get great emotional satisfaction.

These last two figures may seem out of place with the next ones: Laumann's surveys showed that 75 percent of men and 29 percent of women say they always have an orgasm. This means a high percentage of women are not having orgasms or having them only some of the time. Laumann's group was surprised by the findings and concluded that despite the seeming emphasis on orgasm among Americans and the popular idea that frequent orgasms are necessary for a happy sex life, there is "not a strong relationship between having orgasms and having a satisfying sexual life."

Not having an orgasm is not the only sexual problem that women experience much more often than men.

- Thirty-three percent of women say they are not interested in sex, compared with 16 percent of men.
- Twenty-one percent of women say sex is not pleasurable, compared with only 10 percent of men.
- Twenty-four percent of women say they cannot orgasm, compared with 8 percent of men.
- Fifteen percent of women experience pain during intercourse compared with 5 percent of men. In addition, 20 percent of women say they have trouble lubricating, a problem that does not apply to men.

Men do surpass women in having anxiety about performance (18 percent of men versus 11 percent of women) and in climaxing too soon (29 percent of men compared with 10 percent of women).

Why Sexual Fitness Is Important

Sex is a basic human function and need. Frustrations, anxiety, fears, or other concerns about their sexuality can adversely affect all other parts of people's lives. A man who has trouble maintaining an erection may feel inadequate, "less than a man," and become withdrawn in his relationship. If he has a tendency to be aggressive, he may take out his frustrations on his partner. His low self-esteem will likely affect his work as well as his relationships with other people. A woman who has no sex drive may feel there is nothing she can do and may shut down her feelings about sex altogether. Couples who are having trouble conceiving a child are often under a great deal of stress, which can have tremendous negative impact on their relationship as well as on their work and social lives.

Some people have health issues that adversely affect their sexual fitness. Diabetes, for example, is a very common disease that can cause impotence in men and loss of sex drive in women. Women and men with heart disease are sometimes afraid (and often unnecessarily so) to engage in sexual activity for fear they will risk further heart damage or even death. Obesity, a growing problem in the United States, is also a hindrance to sexual fitness in that it can make sexual activity difficult or uncomfortable as well as lower self-esteem.

But people with these and other issues about sexual

functioning can do many things to ameliorate their problems. When it comes to sex, American men and women may be talking about it more than they used to, but there is still very much they do not fully know or understand about it. Once armed with basic information about how the sex organs function and how the mind-body connection is an integral part of sexuality, you can make simple changes in your life that can add more physical, emotional, and spiritual vigor, excitement, and satisfaction to your sexual relationship. This book helps you get that basic knowledge and then shows you how to achieve peak sexual performance, optimal sexual fitness, and new heights of sexual pleasure using natural, nondrug methods.

The Healing Power of Sex

Being as sexually fit as possible not only helps you better enjoy your sexual encounters; it also can improve your overall fitness and health. It's been said that sexual experiences have "a healing power that transcends medicine." The nurturing and healing power of touch has been recognized since ancient times, but only recently has it come under scientific scrutiny. Now experts tell us what people have known intuitively for thousands of years: Touch can heal. Sexual contact is the ultimate touch and so has the highest ability to transform when given with love and tenderness.

Sexual intimacy during and after illness can be an integral part of the recovery process. A person who is recovering from surgery or a heart condition, for example, or individuals who have a chronic condition, such as diabetes or multiple sclerosis, can greatly benefit physically, emotionally, and spiritually from intimacy with their partner. Such intimacy does not need to include sexual intercourse. Many other forms of intimate sexual contact can heal, such as a back rub, a foot massage, mutual masturbation, showering together, or simply cuddling together.

People who are physically challenged may not be able to make love in the conventional sense, but that does not mean they do not enjoy sex. In fact, some disabled people who have lost certain sensations and functions, such as someone who is paralyzed from the waist down, say that other body parts have become more highly sensitized to compensate for the loss of feeling in their genitals.

Sexual activity can help you heal from everyday "hurts." A satisfying sexual experience can help resolve stress and tension, lift your spirits, boost your energy level, and rejuvenate your relationship with your partner. All of these positive benefits, and more, contribute to overall improved sexual fitness and health. It is an empowering state of health to be in, and this book can help you get there.

How This Book Can Help You Achieve Peak Performance

Maintaining sexual fitness is like taking care of your car: You need to perform routine tasks to keep it running at its best. In addition to fueling/feeding your car properly, you need to keep the fluid levels up, change the oil, fill the tires, tune the engine, and dozens of other jobs to keep it running right.

Your body likewise needs maintenance. First you need to know your body's parts and how they work, which is explained in Chapter 2. There are also various lifestyle choices and medical conditions that impact sexual fitness, and these are addressed in Chapter 3. Among the list of "to dos" designed to help maintain the body and keep it operating at an optimal level is proper nutrition, which is discussed in Chapter 4. The power of natural substances from the realms of herbal medicine and homeopathy are explored in Chapter 5, while in Chapter 6 you and your partner can learn how to improve your sexual fitness and performance by doing exercises for couples. Chapter 7 shares some of the sexual secrets from Eastern traditions that are perfect for couples in love, and Chapter 8 reveals how you and your mate can utilize your most important sex organ—your mind—to achieve peak sexual performance and fitness.

Sexual fitness begins with understanding your body—and that of your partner—so you can best experience and enjoy the sexual times you share and know what to do when something doesn't seem right. For many men and women, such knowledge requires a look at an "owner's manual" for the human body. Chapter 2 offers you that look—an overview of a man's and woman's sexual organs and how they operate—or may fail to operate—in the art of lovemaking.

CHAPTER TWO

How Sex Works

If you want to be sexually fit, it's helpful to know how the body parts that are responsible for fitness work. That knowledge can empower you to dispel needless worries about whether something you or your partner is doing or feeling is "normal" or if something may be awry. Understanding how your body functions during sex allows you to relax in the moment and fully share your sexual experience with your partner. It is especially helpful if both you and your partner learn about how sex works for each other. This chapter explains how sexual "parts" consist of much more than just the penis and vagina: A lot of players are working behind the scenes in sexual functioning. It also discusses some basic guidelines for keeping the parts in good health.

What You Know About Sex

When you hear the word "sex," what's the first thought that comes to mind? For many people it is the physical act of sexual intercourse or some other type of sexual intimacy, such as oral sex. As an adult, what you know about sex is the result of what you assimilated from all the information you got as a child and adolescent. But it is never too late to learn something new about sex and about how the human body operates during sexual activity. Many of the fears and anxieties men and women have about their sexual relationships come from ignorance: They do not know or understand what constitutes normal sexual functioning. Perhaps they got wrong information and still think it is true; rather than admit they don't know something, they choose to pretend they do.

Many people believe the media blitz that tells them they need young, "beautiful" bodies, that they should be having earth-moving orgasms, and that everyone who is anyone is enjoying passionate sex all the time. Compounding these distorted expectations even further is the fact that we live in a society that still has trouble talking about sex in a mature fashion.

This chapter brings sex back to basics: what is normal male sexual functioning, what is normal female sexual functioning, and how to ensure that when two people meet—in either a heterosexual or a homosexual relationship—they do so in a way that is satisfying and fulfilling for both partners.

But sex is more than just a physical experience; it is also sensual, emotional, and spiritual. Although the focus of this chapter is on the physical aspect of sexual fitness, these other three components are also incorporated into every sexual act, because they are an integral part of how people respond sexually.

Male Sexual Functioning

Male sexuality begins in the womb. By the twelfth week of pregnancy, the male fetus begins to produce the sex hormone testosterone and its metabolic derivative, dihydrotestosterone. Production stops by week 24 and does not start up again until male children reach puberty, around age 13 or 14. At that time, the hypothalamus and pituitary glands stimulate the testicles to create large amounts of testosterone and a much smaller amount of the female hormone, estrogen. The increase in testosterone production is responsible for sex-related changes such as enlargement of the penis, growth of body hair, deepening voice, and development of scrotal skin folds.

Male Sex Organs

Sexual fitness requires that all parts of the male sexual system work together. These parts include the penis, testes, prostate gland, scrotum, epididymis, vas deferens, urethra, seminal vesicles, and bulbourethral gland. (See Figure 2.1.) Each of these organs has specific functions that are important for sexual arousal and satisfaction as well as for reproduction.

The *penis* is a tube-shaped organ that consists of erectile tissue, blood vessels, and a rich supply of nerve endings concentrated mainly at the tip, which is known as the *glans* or glans penis. The part of the penis that is visible is called the *shaft*. A tube called the *urethra* runs along the entire length of the penis and exits at the glans. The urethra carries semen and urine, but not both at the same time.

When a man becomes sexually aroused, the two types of tissue that surround the urethra become filled with blood—the *corpus spongiosum,* which is on the underside of the penis, and the *corpora cavernosa,* which runs above the corpus spongiosum on both sides of the shaft. The corpus spongiosum is highly sensitive to touch and can be felt when the penis is erect.

Hanging under and behind the penis is the *scrotum,* a pouch of skin that harbors the *testes* (singular, testis), two oval-shaped glands that are the manufacturing centers for sperm. Each testis produces approximately 1,000 sperm per second, or 100 million per day. During ejaculation, a man typically releases between 300 and 500 million sperm.

The scrotum keeps the temperature of the testes about 5 degrees F lower than that of the body's normal temperature of 98.6 degrees F. This lower temperature is critical for production of healthy sperm. When men are in cold surroundings or are sexually excited, the

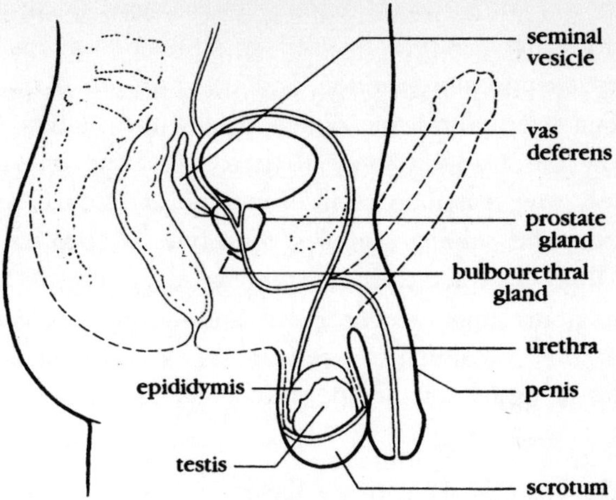

FIGURE 2.1

scrotum moves closer to the body; in a warmer environment, the scrotum hangs away from the body. This allows the testes to remain at a constant temperature.

The testes are also responsible for secretion of a male sex hormone, testosterone. This hormone controls a man's sex drive, stimulates production of sperm, and maintains secondary sex characteristics, such as facial hair.

Sperm is stored in a mass of tightly coiled tubes called the *epididymis,* which sits on top of the testes. When a man becomes sexually aroused and is about to ejaculate, the sperm is set into motion. Two tubes called *vàs deferens* carry the sperm away from the testes to the urethra. Fluids that aid the sperm in its transport are added to it. These fluids come from two sources: the *seminal vesicles,* finger-length organs located behind the bladder; and the *prostate gland,* a walnut-sized gland that wraps around the urethra just below the bladder. Only 10 percent of the approximately one teaspoon of fluid emitted at ejaculation is sperm. The seminal vesicles contribute 60 percent of the fluid in a secretion containing sugar, which provides nourishment to the sperm; and the prostate gland adds the remaining 30 percent as a secretion that makes it easier for the sperm to enter the vagina.

Male Sexual Response Cycle

When men and women become sexually aroused, ideally all of the organs work in a synchronized fashion in a four-stage process called the *sexual response cycle.* Although the names of the stages are the same for both men and women, what occurs during them differs. Here's what happens during the male sexual response cycle.

The first is the *excitement phase.* When a man hears, sees, or otherwise senses something that excites him sexually, the brain sends signals to the penis. The muscles of the penis relax, which allows the corpus spongiosum and corpora cavernosa to fill with blood. As the penis becomes erect, other changes take place: Breathing and heart rate increase, and blood pressure rises.

If sexual excitement continues, the man enters the *plateau phase.* The penis continues to change, becoming fully erect as the glans turns dark red or purple. A drop or two of fluid may appear on the tip of the penis as the bulbourethral glands are activated. The testicles increase in size by as much as 50 percent and draw close to the body.

Internally, the sperm travels from the testicles, through the vas deferens, and to the urethra. Along the way the prostate gland and seminal vesicles add other fluids to the sperm to make up the semen. All of this activity reaches a breaking point known as "ejaculatory inevitability," which means ejaculation occurs even if all stimulation stops.

As a man ejaculates, he enters the *orgasm phase*. During orgasm, which typically lasts between four and ten seconds, the semen is ejected from the penis in a series of three to five contractions. Ejaculation is usually, but not always, accompanied by orgasm. Other bodily responses include an increase in heart rate, blood pressure, and breathing rate, and the toes may curl. Some men have orgasm without ejaculation, which happens among men who have had prostate surgery or those who have a second orgasm within a short time after the first.

The final phase is *resolution,* during which the penis and testicles return to the size they were before sexual stimulation. This part of resolution takes about ten minutes, and during that time the penis is insensitive to stimulation. The other part of the resolution phase is the refractory period, which is the time between ejaculation and being able to have another erection. In younger men this period can be as brief as 15 or 20 minutes; in older men it can be as long as a few days.

Female Sexual Functioning

Female sexuality also begins in the womb around week 12. That's when the external genitalia—the labia minora and labia majora—begin to form. Development of the internal organs then begins, and by week 38, the ovaries have moved into the upper part of the pelvis. This is also the time a female's eggs are formed and stored—between 2 and 4 million immature eggs await the onset of puberty before they have the opportunity to become mature.

During puberty, which usually begins between the ages of 10 and 14, the ovaries are stimulated into action by the secretion of hormones from the pituitary gland. As the ovaries release the female sex hormone estrogen, physical transformations take place, such as breast development, growth of body hair, an increase in height, changes in hair and skin complexion, and the start of the menstrual cycle.

Female sexual functioning is more complex than that of the male because women's bodies are capable of generating, nurturing, and giving birth to new life. As part of this reproductive miracle, women experience the menstrual cycle. The hormones that are involved in the menstrual cycle, including luteinizing hormones, follicle-stimulating hormones, estrogen, and testosterone, play a significant role in the level of a woman's sexual desire, arousal, and satisfaction. Many women, for example, are most sexually responsive during the time their estrogen levels are rising, which is around days 10 to 20 of their menstrual cycle. Then, as their estrogen levels decline, so does the desire for sex.

Female Sexual System

A woman's response to sexual stimulation is not as easy to see as that of a man, because most of a woman's sex organs are internal (see Figure 2.2). The organ most closely associated with sexual pleasure, however, is external. The clitoris is a pea-size organ located above the vaginal opening. It appears to have only one purpose: to provide sexual pleasure. Despite its small size, the clitoris contains as many nerve endings as the head of a penis. When a woman is sexually aroused, the clitoris emerges beyond the skin fold called the *clitorial hood* and becomes erect.

The vaginal opening and the clitoris are protected by two folds of skin, or lips, known as the labia minora (inner lips) and the labia majora (outer lips). The labia majora are usually covered with pubic hair.

Protected within a woman's pelvic cavity are the vagina, cervix, uterus, fallopian tubes, and ovaries. The *vagina* is a muscular tube-shaped organ that has several roles. Although it is only about $3^1/_2$ inches in length, it can expand to receive the penis during intercourse and serve as a passageway for an infant during birth. It is also the organ through which menstrual blood flows as it leaves the body.

When a woman becomes sexually excited, the walls of the vagina expand and become wet with a lubricating fluid. If the fluid reaches the vaginal opening, it will ease penetration by the penis. If it does not, a vaginal lubricant may be needed before intercourse.

About two-thirds up the front side of the vaginal wall is a site known as the *Grafenberg* or *G spot,* named after the gynecologist who first suggested its existence. This dime-size area nearly doubles in size when a woman is sexually aroused. Some women claim that orgasms that result from stimulation of this spot are different from those produced by clitoral stimulation.

At the top of the vagina is the *cervix,* which is the opening into the *uterus,* or womb. A tiny opening in the cervix, called the cervical os, is the doorway through which sperm enters and menstrual blood leaves the uterus. The primary function of the uterus is to nourish a developing fetus. This hollow, pear-shaped organ has an inner lining that thickens each month in anticipation of a fertilized egg. If fertilization does not occur, the lining is shed as the menstrual flow.

Flanking the uterus are the *ovaries,* where the eggs (or ova) are produced. The ovaries also release the hormones estrogen and progesterone. In sexually mature women, many eggs ripen each month, although

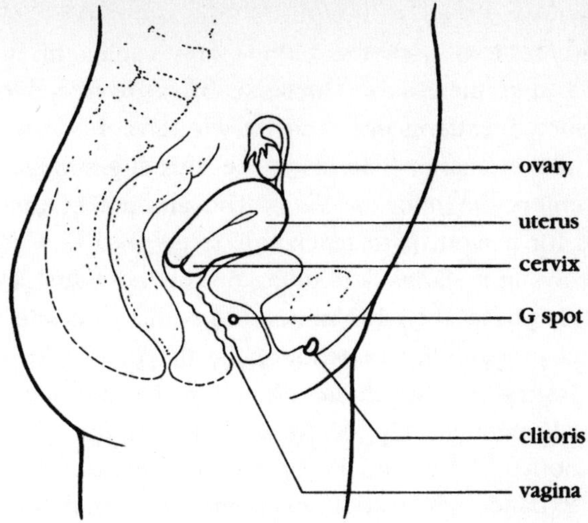

FIGURE 2.2

only one or sometimes a few reach maturity. The body reabsorbs the eggs that do not fully mature.

Female Sexual Response Cycle

As a woman enters the *excitement phase,* the vaginal opening may become wet with a lubricating fluid secreted by the vagina. Lubrication usually begins 10 to 30 seconds after stimulation starts, and it is one of the first signs of sexual excitement in women. Other visible signs include slight enlargement of the breasts, erect nipples, and a darkening of the areolae. Some women also experience a fine rash or reddish hue to the skin, sometimes called a *sex flush*. Internally, the uterus shifts position, both the clitoris and vagina fill with blood, and there is an increase in heart rate, blood pressure, breathing rate, and muscle tension.

If the woman continues to be sexually stimulated, she enters the *plateau phase*. The amount of time it takes for a woman to reach this stage, and how long she stays in it, varies depending on the individual. During this phase, the labia minora fill with blood and the vagina prepares for penetration by the penis. To help this process, the *vestibular glands*, which are near the vaginal opening, may secrete a lubricating fluid. To accommodate the penis, the upper two thirds of the vagina expands while the lower third grows narrower to better grip the penis during intercourse.

The sexual tension that has been growing during the excitement and plateau phases is released during the *orgasm phase*. An orgasm is a series of contractions, or spasms, in the genitals, although other parts of the body, or indeed the entire body, may respond during this phase. Orgasm usually lasts 10 to 15 seconds and is a highly individual experience. Some women moan, cry out, arch their back, and clutch the sheets or their partner; others are quiet and still. Curled toes and dilated pupils are common responses, as are muscle twitches in the legs.

Women differ greatly from men in this phase because unlike men, who can have only one type of orgasm, women can experience four: those that result from stimulation of the clitoris, the G spot, or a combination of the two; and multiple orgasms. Some women, however, rarely or never experience orgasm. Many experts believe that many women who find it difficult or impossible to achieve orgasm during sexual intercourse can learn to do so, through sensate focus exercises and masturbation. (See Chapter 7.)

As the contractions of orgasm fade away, the *resolution phase* begins. This is when the body returns to the pre-excitement phase, a process that takes a few minutes. The genital area takes longer—usually 30 minutes or more. If, however, sexual stimulation continues, a woman may return to the plateau phase and move into the orgasm phase again and again until she finally enters resolution. Some women report feeling a sexual "afterglow" of overall body warmth or tingling, or a feeling of euphoria for several hours after orgasm.

What About Foreplay?

Foreplay is a commonly used term that refers to the sexual activity that precludes sexual intercourse, notably during the excitement phase and into the plateau phase. Sex researchers William Masters, M.D., and Virginia Johnson of the Masters and Johnson Institute in St. Louis object to the term because they feel it comes with expectations: It implies that the kissing, stroking, massaging, and other stimulating activities are steps people "have to do" or are expected to do in order to reach the goal, which is intercourse. Masters and Johnson prefer the term "noncoital sex play," which removes the expectation and pressure to perform associated with the term "foreplay."

It is just as important to be sexually fit for noncoital sex play as it is for sexual intercourse. In fact, you can easily make sexual fitness into sex play, and vice versa. The couples exercises in Chapter 6 and the massage techniques discussed in Chapter 8 are good preludes to a romantic interlude that may or may not include sexual intercourse.

If you and your partner do move on to sexual intercourse, beware of the "mad dash" to the finish. Research shows that men tend to rush through foreplay to get to the "good part" while women want more sex play. If both partners want to reach orgasm, then the woman usually needs more of the right type of stimulation. Dr. Alfred Kinsey, author of the Kinsey reports on sexual behavior, noted that it is harder for women to reach orgasm through intercourse than it is through masturbation. This is true, he said, because although women generally have the ability to reach orgasm as quickly as men do, men often do not provide the type of stimulation women need to do so.

The solution is communication. Sexual partners need to tell each other, either verbally or in another way, what is sexually stimulating for them. An excellent way to learn new sexual communication skills is to practice Eastern sexual exercises, like those explained in Chapter 7.

Orgasm

So much mystery and misinformation surrounds orgasm, or the "big O," that it deserves special consideration. Most of the questions surround a woman's orgasm, because a man's orgasm is much more straightforward. Men should read on, however, as they can use the information to enhance their sexual relationship.

For some couples orgasm is the goal of their sexual encounter; it is a measure of their sexual fitness and aptitude. For others it is desirable but not essential. About 10 percent of women have never had an orgasm. At least another 20 percent have an orgasm only occasionally. If you take the anxiety out of wondering whether you will experience an orgasm or if your partner will feel inadequate if you do not have an orgasm, you can improve your sexual fitness and your relationship. You can begin by better understanding what orgasm is and is not.

- Orgasm is a deeply personal experience, and people can experience orgasm differently each time, depending on their mood, stress level, type and amount of foreplay, relationship with their partner, and energy level. For women, for example, the time of the month and the corresponding hormone levels can change the way the uterus contracts during arousal and thus change the orgasm experience.

• Not every sexual experience results in orgasm, especially for women. Sexual satisfaction does not depend on having an orgasm.

• Although sex researchers have not clearly established the source of a woman's orgasm (the clitoris, the G spot, the mind, or all three), some women can reach orgasm just by thinking erotic thoughts.

• Although it may feel as if orgasm begins in the genitals, it is actually controlled by the hypothalamus and limbic system in the brain. This fact supports the theory that orgasm originates in the mind.

• Simultaneous orgasm is a goal of many couples, but reaching it can so occupy the thoughts of some partners that they forget to enjoy sex and each other.

• Faking orgasm is common: As many as 20 percent of women fake orgasm at least occasionally, if not always. Most do it to prevent their partner from feeling inadequate. Women who have difficulty achieving orgasm can benefit from practicing sensate focus exercises (see Chapter 6) or masturbation.

Masturbation

Masturbation is self-stimulation for sexual pleasure, often to the point of orgasm. It is a sexual practice most men and women, married and single, do at least occasionally, yet many of them do not admit it. It can play a significant role in sexual fitness, as masturbation can help both men and women learn about their own normal sexual functioning and sexual desires as well as what their partner likes. In women, it helps keep the vagina toned.

Masturbation as Therapy

Many sex therapists prescribe masturbation for women who have trouble reaching orgasm. These women need to become comfortable with themselves and pay close attention to what triggers sexual response in them. They can then tell or guide their partner to do the same thing for them, or simply use what they've learned to please themselves.

Masturbation is also a good way to keep the vaginal tissues pliable and moist. Women who are postmenopausal often experience dry vaginal tissues, which masturbation can remedy.

For men who experience premature ejaculation, carefully controlled masturbation exercises can help cure this problem. See Chapter 6 for instructions.

Some couples practice mutual masturbation, which can be a way to heighten sexual excitement and pleasure as well as an alternative to sexual intercourse, especially for individuals who may have limited mobility or strength because of a physical condition. Mutual masturbation has gained acceptance among many people now as a safe sexual activity because of the threat of AIDS. (For more information about masturbation, including techniques, see Suggested Readings.)

Still Taboo

Masturbation remains a hush-hush topic, associated with guilt, shame, and embarrassment. Yet this natural activity, when practiced in privacy and for purposes of pleasure and/or sexual healing, can be very effective and satisfying. It is a problem only when it is done to excess, which can perhaps be best defined as masturbation that becomes addictive and disrupts a person's lifestyle. This occurs in a very small percentage of people and usually can be remedied with therapy.

Basic Sexual Fitness Guidelines

Knowing how you and your partner's sexual parts work is only part of the story of sexual fitness; the other part is keeping them healthy. The following basic sexual fitness guidelines can have a tremendous impact on your sexual and overall health.

Genital Cleanliness

The market is flooded with deodorant and cosmetic products that the manufacturers say are needed to get and stay clean and fresh. Many people, especially women, believe that their natural body smells are unhealthy or unnatural and need to be eliminated. But when it comes to the genital area, it is possible to be too clean.

Many producers of feminine hygiene products send the message that the natural smell of a woman's vagina and vulva is unpleasant. Yet the natural scents and secretions of a woman's genital area are an important factor in sexual arousal and desire as well as sexual health. The vagina and labia have sensitive tissues that provide an environment for a specific pH level and a home for "good," or healthy, bacteria. This delicate balance of pH and bacteria can be upset by factors such as douching, the use of bubble bath or bath salts, application of feminine deodorant sprays, washing with scented soaps, and wearing synthetic underwear. These and other factors allow the growth of unhealthy bacteria and open the door to the possibility of vaginal bacterial and yeast infections.

Women can keep their genital area clean by using plain water for the vulval area and unscented soap and water for the anal area. For women who feel they need to use soap on their vulval region, unscented soap is recommended, and thorough rinsing is important to prevent infection. Douching a healthy vagina can actually encourage yeast infections.

Cleanliness for men is also simple. Plain water is generally sufficient, although a mild, unscented soap also may be used. Uncircumcised men should wash under the foreskin daily; circumcised men should wash the glans every day. All men need to use soap and water to clean the anal area daily.

Undergarments

Underwear made of synthetic fibers such as polyester or nylon promote sweating, which in turn stimulates the growth of bacteria and yeast. Both men and women need to wear cotton or silk underwear, which allows for air circulation. Women who wear pantyhose should buy brands that have a cotton crotch. Men who wear tight briefs or tight jeans are susceptible to low sperm counts because the scrotum is brought close to the body, which raises the temperature in the scrotum and kills the sperm.

The sheer force of gravity makes breasts of any size sag eventually, which is why it is recommended that women wear a bra. The ligaments responsible for holding up breasts are not very strong, and they quickly lose their elasticity, especially when breasts are large. Wearing a bra reduces the amount of stress on the ligaments. There are also exercises you can do to firm up the muscles under the breasts.

Routine Examinations

Routine checkups are essential if you want to maintain sexual and overall health. For women, a yearly gynecological examination, which includes a Pap smear and pelvic examination, is recommended. A yearly or biyearly mammogram is generally recommended beginning at age 40. Beginning at age 16, women are encouraged to do monthly breast self-examinations, preferably just after the end of a menstrual period. A breast examination is often included with the yearly pelvic examination.

For men, a testicular self-examination should be done every month to detect any lumps or swelling that may indicate cancer. These tests should begin at about age 14 to 16. Beginning at age 40, doctors recommend that men have a yearly prostate examination.

Testing for sexually transmitted diseases (see Chapter 3) is recommended for any man or woman who has symptoms of these conditions or who has had casual sex and is concerned he or she may have contracted a disease.

Safer Sex

Few things can put more of a damper on sexual activity than contracting a sexually transmitted disease (STD). (See Chapter 3.) Of major concern are HIV, or the human immunodeficiency virus, and AIDS, or acquired immunodeficiency syndrome, which affect both men and women, heterosexual and homosexual, as well as children, and which have a high mortality rate. Two diseases in particular—chlamydia and gonorrhea—are an especial threat to women's fertility as well as a threat to the health of any infant that may be born to an infected mother.

To significantly reduce the risk of transmitting or getting such a condition, people who engage in vaginal or anal sex are encouraged to use latex condoms. This practice is especially recommended among high-risk groups, such as people who have casual sex, have multiple sex partners, or who have sex with an infected partner. A substance called nonoxynol-9, which kills bacteria and viruses, including HIV, should be used with condoms.

Before you have sex with someone for the first time, have a frank discussion about your sexual histories. For extra safety, do it with the lights on. For women, this will allow you to see if there are any signs of disease, such as sores or bumps on the penis, signs of inflammation, or unusual discharge from the end of the penis. Signs of STDs often are not apparent in women.

If you have any reason to believe you may have a sexually transmitted disease, see your physician immediately or go to a clinic and ask for a full battery of tests for STDs.

Sex, like life, does not always run smoothly. Sometimes sexual functioning goes awry, temporarily or permanently. The next chapter examines some of the more common challenges to sexual fitness and sexual health.

CHAPTER THREE

When Sexual Function Goes Awry

Sex is a many splendored and multifaceted experience that involves a complex exchange of messages between the mind and body, glands and hormones, and various organs systems as well as communication, spoken and unspoken, between partners. In addition, there are inner stressors—such as fluctuating hormone levels, poor diet, heredity factors—and outer ones—such as relationship problems, job tension, and environmental pollutants. It's no wonder, then, that the mind-body sometimes rebels, and that rebellion often has a detrimental effect on sexual energy and fitness.

When sexual function goes awry, it can show up as impotence, loss of sexual desire, painful intercourse, infertility, or premature ejaculation. All of these problems may have one or more causes, which are related to lifestyle, medical conditions, or both.

Lifestyle, such as poor nutrition, insufficient sleep,

exposure to environmental toxins, emotional and physical stress, and use of alcohol or drugs, both legal and illegal, can have a negative effect on sexual function. Likewise, medical conditions and life stages, such as cardiovascular disease, diabetes, arthritis, sexually transmitted diseases, lung disease, menopause, and aging, can cause sexual difficulties and detract from sexual fitness.

This chapter discusses the different sexual dysfunctions and the stressors that can cause or contribute to them. Each discussion includes natural remedy suggestions that you can explore elsewhere in this book.

Types of Sexual Dysfunction

Impotence

The inability to get or maintain an erection that is sufficient for penetration and ejaculation three out of four times (75 percent) is defined as clinical impotence, or erectile dysfunction. Estimates as to the number of men who experience impotence varies, with some experts saying that approximately 30 million men in the United States have this problem. It is estimated that 55 percent of men will experience erectile dysfunction by the time they reach age 75.

Eighty-five percent of cases of impotence have a physical cause, such as atherosclerosis, alcohol and drug use, prostate disorders, hypertension, stroke, low levels of testosterone (male sex hormone) and/or high levels of estrogen (female sex hormone), diabetes, multiple sclerosis, hypothyroidism, and neurological disorders. About 10 percent are attributed to psychological problems, such as depression, stress, and performance anxiety, while about 5 percent have unknown causes.

If you are experiencing impotence, it is recommended that you first get an examination by a physician to determine if a medical condition is causing the problem. Atherosclerosis (hardening of the artery walls) of the penile artery is the main cause of impotence among all cases and in about 50 percent of men older than 50 years. Atherosclerosis can be reversed; proper diet (see Chapter 4) that emphasizes whole, low-fat foods, along with lifestyle practices that include stress reduction and exercise and restriction of alcohol have been proven to dramatically reverse blocked arteries.

The Association for Male Sexual Dysfunction has identified more than 200 drugs that may cause impotence. Many of these are prescription drugs, especially those designed to lower blood pressure (diuretics, calcium channel blockers, angiotensin-converting enzyme inhibitors, and beta blockers). Others include antidepressants, narcotics, sedatives, antihistamines, and alcohol. If you are taking a prescription medication and are impotent, consult with your physician or pharmacist. In many cases a natural approach (diet, exercise, herbs, nutritional supplements) can replace the prescription and may eliminate impotence.

Natural remedies to treat either the physical or emotional causes of impotence include nutritional supplements and some foods (pumpkin seeds, avocado, sesame seeds, zinc; see Chapter 4); herbs (ashwagandha, brier, cinnamon, ginseng, lycium fruit, potency wood, pygeum, sarsasparilla, saw palmetto, yohimbe) and homeopathy (agnus, conium, lycopodium; see Chapter 5).

Infertility: His and Hers

Infertility in humans is defined as the inability to conceive after 18 to 24 months of routine, unprotected sexual intercourse. Infertility affects approximately 10 to 15 percent of married couples, and the "blame" is evenly split: 40 percent of the time it is due to a female factor and 40 percent of cases are due to a male factor. Up to 35 percent of these couples must deal with more than one cause. The cause in 20 percent of all cases remains a mystery.

Causes of female infertility can be placed into three categories: failure to ovulate, inability of the egg and sperm to unite, and inability of the uterus to support and nurture a growing fetus. Each category in turn has several causes, which demonstrates how complex the issue of infertility can be. In most cases, however, infertility can be treated, although not always naturally. Blocked fallopian tubes, for example, may need to be opened surgically. Failure to ovulate sometimes can be remedied with herbal or homeopathic formulas.

According to the World Health Organization, one in

15 men is infertile. The most common cause of infertility in men is a low sperm count. For a male to be fertile, the sperm must meet the following criteria: more than 20 million sperm per milliliter of semen; more than 50 percent of the sperm must be able to swim effectively; and more than 50 percent of the sperm must be of normal shape. Male infertility is on the rise, and many experts believe environmental toxins are a significant cause. Some chemicals, such as those found in paints, herbicides, and adhesives, can cause a low sperm count. Other factors that lead to a low sperm count are varicocele (swollen veins in the scrotum), obesity, smoking, alcohol abuse, a diet that is poor in vitamins and minerals, stress, and treatment with drugs such as chemotherapy.

Natural approaches to infertility in men include various foods and nutritional supplements (essential fatty acids, zinc, vitamins E and B6; see Chapter 4); herbs (damiana, ginseng, pygeum, saw palmetto; see Chapter 5); and mind-body methods (see Chapter 8). Women can use the same foods and supplements as recommended for men; they also can try herbs (garlic, agnus castus, skullcap; see Chapter 5); and mind-body methods (see Chapter 8).

Lack of Sexual Desire: His and Hers

Both men and women can experience low sex drive or lack of sexual desire. For centuries, the idea that it was natural for women to have a sex drive didn't occur to most people because women were expected to just "lie there" and do their "marital duty" when it came to sex. Fortunately those days are gone, but in their place has come the realization that lack of or low sexual desire is a common problem among women. For many women the cause is emotional, associated with past physical and/or emotional abuse issues, societal expectations, relationship problems, and stress. Physical factors, such as low hormone levels, drug use, nutritional deficiencies, or pain during sex (see "Painful Intercourse," p. 39) also may play a part.

Men can also experience a diminished sex drive, which is usually associated with stress around their work, relationship, health, or financial status. Occasionally it is caused by past abuse issues, fear of intimacy, or low self-esteem.

One other cause of a low sex drive among men has recently received much attention. "A relative excess of estrogen to testosterone dampens down male sexuality," says Eugene Shippen, M.D., author of *The Testosterone Syndrome: The Critical Factor for Energy, Health, & Sexuality—Reversing the Male Menopause*. Extra estrogen can hinder the effectiveness of the testosterone that is in the body as well as increase a man's risk for heart disease.

Natural ways to remedy lack of sexual desire include some foods and nutritional supplements (cruciferous vegetables and soy products; L-phenylalanine and tyrosine, histidine, DHEA, bee pollen, essential fatty acids; see Chapter 4); herbs and herbal formulas (agnus castus, ashwagandha, catuaba, cinnamon, dong quai, ginseng, oats, potency wood, saw palmetto, schisandra berries, yohimbe; see Chapter 5); homeopathic remedies (causticum, phosphoric acid, sepia); and mind-body methods (see Chapter 8).

Painful Intercourse: His and Hers

For some women every sexual experience is a physically painful one. Painful sex, or dyspareunia, can be caused by lack of lubrication (often associated with menopause), a vaginal or pelvic infection such as pelvic inflammatory disease (PID), sexually transmitted disease, or endometriosis, or it can stem from anger, fear, or tension. The cause of the pain should be determined by a gynecologist if the origin seems to be physical or by a sex therapist if the source is emotional.

A type of painful sex that is caused by an involuntary tightening of the vaginal muscles or spastic contractions of the muscles at the vaginal opening is called *vaginismus*. Women who have this dysfunction are generally extremely afraid or anxious about sexual intercourse but may not consciously recognize the reason why. Work with a sex therapist or counselor, along with some exercises to help relax the vaginal muscles (see Chapter 6), can resolve the situation.

Men also can experience painful intercourse, which typically occurs as painful ejaculation. This condition usually is caused by prostatitis or an inflamed prostate gland. (See "Prostatic and Testicular Conditions," p. 57.)

Natural approaches to ease or resolve painful intercourse include the following remedies: nutritional supplements (vitamins A and E, acidophilus; see Chapter 4); homeopathy (apis, aurum metallicum, belladonna, calcarea, sepia; see Chapter 5); and exercises to relax the vagina (see Chapter 6).

Premature Ejaculation

Premature ejaculation, which is ejaculation either before or soon after the penis achieves penetration, affects approximately 30 percent of men. In nearly all cases it is psychological in origin, with performance anxiety being the most common cause. Premature ejaculation can be treated naturally with various herbal, homeopathic, and nutritional remedies designed to relieve tension and anxiety, and by specific exercises. Avoidance of caffeine and other stimulants is recommended. Natural remedies and supplements include the following: herbs (damiana, ginseng, lycium fruit, skullcap, valerian) and homeopathy (lycopodium, nux vomica, graphites; see Chapter 5). Several easy methods used to treat premature ejaculation are described in Chapter 6, and Eastern approaches are in Chapter 7.

Special Exercises

The following special exercise techniques can help you and your partner correct and heal several different conditions that can limit your sexual fitness. Also see Chapter 7 for special exercises done according to the Eastern tradition, Taoism.

Treating Premature Ejaculation

When a man is feeling highly aroused and is about to ejaculate but to do so would be premature, his partner can use two squeeze methods and a stop-start technique to postpone ejaculation.

- Top Squeeze Method: Grasp the penis by placing the thumb on the underside where the head and shaft meet and positioning two or three fingers on the opposite side of the shaft. Apply firm pressure for 10 to 20 seconds, until the feeling of intense arousal fades. Do not move your fingers, because the slightest movement may stimulate ejaculation.
- Bottom Squeeze Method: Use the same grip and method as explained above, only apply it at the base of the penis.
- Stop-Start Technique: This technique has three stages, which provide the best results when done in order. In stage 1, the man's partner masturbates the penis until just before an impending

ejaculation, then stops to allow the urge to subside. This should be repeated at least three times before the man allows himself to ejaculate. In stage 2, the same method is followed, only this time a lubricant should be used. Once the man is comfortable with these two stages, he is ready for intercourse. The woman-on-top position is recommended at this point. Just before ejaculation is imminent, the man should signal to his partner so she can stop and allow the urgent feeling to subside before starting again. This sequence should be repeated three times before the man allows himself to ejaculate.

Reducing Painful Intercourse for Women

- Use a hand mirror to examine your genitals. Part the lips of your vulva gently.
- Locate the entrance into your vagina with the tip of your index finger. (Make sure your fingernail is cut short!)
- Lubricate your finger with saliva, K-Y jelly, or another lubricant gel. Gently insert the tip of your index finger into your vagina. As you do, bear down, as if you were trying to push your fingertip out. This action loosens the vaginal muscles.
- Keep your fingertip in your vagina for a few minutes. Focus on how it feels. As you get

used to the feeling, move your finger in a little farther.

- Tighten your vaginal muscles around your finger, then relax. Repeat this exercise several times. If you feel relaxed, insert your finger in a bit farther each time you tighten and release.
- Once you are comfortable up to this step, try inserting two fingers. Tighten and relax as you did above.
- Practice this exercise until you are ready for your partner to insert his finger. Use a lubricant.
- Once you and your partner can reach this point in the exercise, try intercourse with the woman-on-top position. This allows the woman control over the depth of penetration.

Pain-Relieving Power of Sex

If menstrual cramps or chronic pain conditions such as arthritis or low-back pain make the thought of sexual activity unappealing, sex may be exactly what the doctor ordered. Studies show that a woman's threshold for pain increases during masturbation. Experts suggest the same effect is possible during lovemaking. Cultures in the East have long known about the pain-relieving powers of sex. In fact, Tantric and Taoist lovemaking exercises and practices were developed to facilitate sexual healing. See Chapter 7 for a discussion of these exercises.

Roadblocks to Sexual Fitness

Alcohol

Consumption of alcohol has many unpleasant side effects on sexual fitness. Although one or two occasional drinks may lower your inhibitions and make you feel more at ease or "sexy," even such small amounts of alcohol can have a suppressive effect, depending on the person. In men, two to three shots of liquor can cause delayed ejaculation and mildly suppressed erections. Higher amounts of alcohol consumption cause many men to experience significant problem with erections. In women, two to three shots of liquor can result in a significant reduction in vaginal blood flow, a longer time to reach orgasm, and a less intense orgasm. The toxins in alcohol cause the testes to shrink, testosterone production to decline, and estrogen levels to rise, which can lead to impotence.

Among serious drinkers, alcohol takes a significant toll. According to Masters and Johnson and to Kolodny, 40 to 50 percent of male alcoholics have little or no sex drive. Thirty to 40 percent of female alcoholics have trouble with sexual arousal, and about 15 percent have little or no ability to reach orgasm or have orgasms that are greatly reduced in frequency and intensity. Alcohol consumption also depletes the body of zinc, a nutrient that is vital for sexual fitness. (See Chapter 4.)

Drugs

Over-the-counter, prescription, and street drugs can all have a detrimental effect on sexual fitness. Antihistamines, for example, used to treat hay fever and colds, can inhibit vaginal lubrication. Antihypertensives, used to treat high blood pressure (hypertension), can cause impotence and decreased sexual desire in men and orgasmic difficulties in women. Between 20 and 25 percent of men who take diuretics can expect to experience impotence and decreased sexual desire.

The box on page 46 lists examples of drugs that have an adverse effect on sexual function and fitness.

Environmental Toxins

More and more scientists are convinced that the poisons being dumped into the air, water, and soil are causing a multitude of health problems, including sexual ones. Since the mid-1970s, male sperm counts have been declining by about 2 percent each year, and the incidence of testicular cancer is rising. Some chemicals, such as those found in paints, inks, adhesives, food packaging, pesticides, and herbicides, are believed to mimic the female hormone estrogen. When these chemicals enter a man's body, they cause the testicles to produce fewer sperm.

At this time, the best defense is avoidance of chemicals as much as possible. Drinking pure water, eating whole, organic foods, avoiding use of pesticides and herbicides in your home and on your lawn, and ensuring that your work environment is safe from environmental toxins are steps you can take to help maintain your health. (See Appendix A for organizations that can pro-

---

DRUGS AND THEIR EFFECTS ON SEXUAL FUNCTION
(Generic Names Given)

ANTIDEPRESSANTS (impotence, loss of desire, ejaculation problems): clomipramine, fluoxetine, phenelzine, sertraline

ANTIEPILEPTIC DRUGS (loss of desire, impotence): carbamazepine, phenobarbital, phenytoin, primidone

ANTIHYPERTENSIVES (impotence): bendroflumethiazide, chlorothiazide, chlorthalidone, spironolactone, propranolol, clonidine, methyldopa, guanethidine, reserpine

ANTIPSYCHOTICS (impotence, ejaculation problems, priapism): clozapine, fluphenazine, haloperidol, perphenazine, thioridazine, trifluoperazine

HORMONES (loss of desire, impotence, ejaculation problems). anabolic steroids, cyproterone, medroxyprogesterone

MISCELLANEOUS DRUGS (loss of desire, impotence): cancer chemotherapy agents, cimetidine, digoxin, ketoconazole

STREET DRUGS (loss of desire, impotence, ejaculation problems): heroin, methadone, morphine, PCP

---

vide more information about environmental toxins; see Suggested Readings for books on detoxifying your life.)

Nicotine

It is well known that tobacco smoking has adverse effects on general health, but did you know that it also reduces the number of viable sperm? Men who smoke and who want to help ensure their fertility need to quit. Smoking also has been associated with impotence. A strong blood flow is essential for getting and maintaining a rigid erection, but smoking reduces blood circulation, which can result in erection problems. Smoking also reduces lung capacity and oxygen flow, both of which are detrimental to overall health and sexual health in particular.

Past Sexual Trauma

For some men and, more often, women, sexual abuse or rape during childhood and/or adulthood has significantly hampered their ability to enjoy intimate sexual relationships. Their feelings about their past can range from anger, fear, and anxiety to shame and guilt. Often these individuals have no interest in sex (and may, in some cases, avoid all intimate contact) or endure painful intercourse caused by their aversion to sex. Counseling is recommended to help overcome the scars left by these experiences.

Stress

The body responds to stress by sending a chemical called adrenaline into the bloodstream. The body can handle this alteration in chemical balance for short periods of time. When stress is chronic, however, the mind-body rebels, and sexual function is one area that suffers. Loss of sexual desire, impotence, and performance anxiety often are associated with stress.

Effective ways to heal the mind-body rebellion are discussed in Chapter 8. Massage, qigong (a Chinese practice combining movement, breathing, and meditation), yoga, and sensate focus exercises are all ways to reduce and eliminate harmful stress and then revive and maintain the mind-body connection in sexual fitness.

Medical Conditions That Challenge Sexual Fitness

We are all sexual beings, and the vast majority of us seek and desire some sexual activity whether we have a medical condition that affects our sexual fitness or not. Continuing or resuming sexual activity during or after an illness, if possible, is a very positive way to reaffirm your life force and your relationship.

As the result of an illness or surgery, you may need to make changes in the ways you make love because your body has new limitations or because of effects of medication. This may be the time to explore new ways to please each other sexually or to share intimate times together in creative ways.

Many medical conditions can present some sort of challenge to sexual functioning, and it is not possible to cover all of them here. The ones to be described represent both the more common ones and those that have a significant impact on sexual activity. Also, if you are taking any medications for a specific problem, they may have a detrimental effect on your sexual functioning. In most cases natural remedies and methods can help you overcome or better cope with the challenges to sexual fitness you may face if you have, for example, diabetes, high blood pressure, or herpes. However, it is not within the scope of this book to offer treatment recommendations for these medical problems. Some exceptions have been made for conditions that involve the reproductive system—dysmenorrhea, menopause, pelvic inflammatory disease, prostate problems, and sexually transmitted diseases.

If you find it difficult to talk with your physician about sexual issues or if he or she is not comfortable with the topic, ask the doctor or nurse to recommend a sex therapist or counselor who can help you. Support groups targeted for specific conditions, such as breast cancer support groups or those for people with herpes, can provide priceless support, advice, and understanding as well. (See Appendix A for a list of support organizations.)

Arthritis

More than 31 million people have some type of the rheumatic diseases known collectively as *arthritis*. The stiff, swollen joints that characterize arthritis can make lovemaking painful and restrict mobility. But sexual activity does not need to cease just because one or both partners have arthritis. In fact, studies show that sexual activity can result in up to six hours of relief from pain.

If you or your partner, or both, have arthritis, try the "spoon" (side-by-side) sexual position to reduce weight-bearing. If you have access to a private pool, try making love in well-heated water. Share a soak in a warm bath. You may want to try a gentle massage (see Chapter 8) with an aromatic essential oil. To enhance your sexual fitness, make appropriate aerobic exercise (swimming, water aerobics, or bicycling; see Chapter 6) a routine part of your lifestyle. Based on your abilities, consider some of the other exercises explained in Chapter 7.

Cancer

Cancer takes both a physical and emotional toll on a patient and his or her partner. Depression, fear, and whatever physical limitations are caused by the cancer or the therapy are issues that need to be dealt with by both parties. Women who have had a mastectomy for breast cancer, for example, have to cope with the loss of one or both breasts and how it makes them feel as sexual beings. A loving, supportive partner is vital for the healing process to be successful. Sex therapists who specialize in recuperative sex therapy are especially helpful in these situations, as are breast cancer support groups.

Some chemotherapy drugs cause loss of libido, inability to reach orgasm, lack of lubrication, and impotence. These effects are irreversible in some cases, as the chemicals permanently reduce sex hormone levels.

Cardiovascular Disease

Many diseases fall into the category of cardiovascular disease, including arrhythmia, angina, and arteriosclerosis. Although many heart patients are afraid to have sex for fear they will suffer another attack or a setback in their recovery, the American Heart Association says that unless patients have been told otherwise by their physician, they can resume sexual activity as soon as they feel they are ready.

A common factor among people with a heart condition is fatigue, so the best time for lovemaking may be in the morning or early afternoon, when they are less tired. As a precaution, heart patients should wait at least two hours after eating before having sex.

If you notice a loss of libido or problems with impotence, premature ejaculation, or lack of vaginal lubrication and you are taking medications for your heart condition, check with your doctor or pharmacist for the side effects of the drugs. Many drugs prescribed for cardiovascular conditions cause sexual difficulties. The most common side effect of beta blockers, for example, is impotence. Both loss of sex drive and impotence are associated with use of ACE (angiotensin converting enzyme) inhibitors and diuretics.

The sexual-fitness exercises described in Chapter 6 and the Eastern sexual exercises in Chapter 7 are generally safe for heart patients. *Always check with your physician before starting any new fitness, nutrition, or supplement program.* To help boost the mind-body sexual connection, also refer to the methods in Chapter 8.

Depression

Clinical depression can have a profound effect on a person's physical, emotional, social, and sexual well-being. It is characterized by feelings of hopelessness, inadequacy, melancholy, and sometimes thoughts of suicide. Depressed individuals often lose interest in common activities, such as eating, socializing, and sex. Clinical depression differs from a depressed mood, which refers to feelings of sadness or "the blues" that last for a short time and do not adversely affect a person's ability to function sexually.

Depression and loss of sexual desire is a chicken-or-the-egg situation. In some cases a person becomes clinically depressed and loss of libido is one of the results; in others a person has a sexual condition, such as impotence, and becomes increasingly despondent and feels worthless and rejected to the point of clinical depression.

People with clinical depression and problems with sexual functioning need to seek the help of a qualified mental health professional who is knowledgeable in sexual issues. (See Appendix A for assistance in locating such individuals.)

Diabetes

Diabetes is a disease in which the body is unable to produce any or enough insulin or to process it properly. It is estimated that approximately 16 million Americans have diabetes, and about half of them are undiagnosed.

Of the two primary types of diabetes—Type I and Type II—about 85 percent have the latter. People with Type I diabetes (insulin-dependent), which usually first occurs in childhood or adolescence, do not produce insulin and require daily medication. Those with Type II (non–insulin-dependent), which usually first appears in people 40 years and older, can be controlled by diet and exercise, medication, or both. Diabetes can have a far-reaching effect on nearly every system in the body, including the neurological, hormonal, and vascular functions.

High blood-sugar levels can lead to various complications, including disruption in hormone production as well as damage to nerves, which leads to impotence and loss of sexual response. Impotence is one of the most common complications of diabetes. Others include limited blood flow to the sex organs, which may occur due to blood vessel damage, or atherosclerotic vascular disease; and damage to the kidneys and nervous system.

Holistic treatments of diabetes include proper diet and an exercise routine, herbal and homeopathic remedies, and stress reduction. (See Suggested Readings for books on holistic treatment of diabetes.)

Dysmenorrhea

Painful menstruation, or dysmenorrhea, is one of the most common menstrual problems women encounter. Symptoms include a dull or sharp pain in the lower back and lower abdomen, headache, diarrhea, and sweating. Two types of dysmenorrhea occur, and both have similar symptoms. Women with primary dysmenorrhea have either an increased level of prostaglandin (a substance that causes uterine contractions) or a higher sensitivity to it. Secondary dysmenorrhea usually begins three or more years after a woman has begun menstruation and may be caused by a pelvic infection, fibroids, stress, endometriosis, or a thyroid problem.

Natural remedies for dysmenorrhea include various foods and supplements (e.g., beets, vitamin B6, bioflavonoids; see Chapter 4); herbal formulas (caraway, cramp bark, catnip, dong quai, peppermint) and homeopathic remedies (chamomilla, colocynthis, belladonna, lycopodium, pulsatilla, nux vomica; see Chapter

5); and mind-body methods (yoga, qigong, massage; see Chapter 8).

Menopause

The cessation of menstruation and of a woman's ability to bear children is known as *menopause*. It can be accompanied by many or few symptoms, which are the result of the sharp decline in estrogen levels that occurs with menopause. Up to 25 percent of menopausal women experience painful intercourse. Some other common symptoms include hot flushes, fatigue, depression, back pain, dry skin, dry hair, incontinence, osteoporosis, insomnia, poor memory, and increased hair growth on the face, stomach, or chest. These symptoms can leave many women feeling little or no interest in sex, at least while they are going through this phase of life.

Some natural remedies to relieve the symptoms of menopause and help revitalize sexual fitness during this stage of life include nutritional supplements (magnesium, selenium, zinc, and vitamin B-complex; see Chapter 4); and herbal and homeopathic remedies (agnus castus, black cohosh, dong quai, ginseng, sepia, valerian; see Chapter 5).

Obesity

Obesity is associated with lower testosterone levels and increased estrogen levels—the formula for male impotence. Being overweight also may sap the amount of energy you have for sexual activity, limit the positions you can use, or inhibit your arousal level.

If you are overweight, begin a healthy weight-loss and exercise program. The dietary guidelines in Chapter 4 are designed for good overall and sexual health and can form the basis of a weight-loss program. (See Suggested Readings for information on a healthy weight-loss program.)

Pelvic Inflammatory Disease

Pelvic inflammatory disease, or PID, is a general term for several inflammatory and infectious conditions that affect the female reproductive system and often cause sexual difficulties. Some of the more common PIDs include vaginitis (vaginal infection, including yeast infection [*Candida*]), endometriosis (growths on the outside of the uterus), and salpingitis (inflammation of the fallopian tubes).

Symptoms of acute PID include painful intercourse, vaginal bleeding after sex, fever with shaking, severe lower abdominal pain, and back pain. Chronic PID can lead to reduced fertility. If you suspect you have PID, consult your physician. Left untreated, PIDs can keep recurring. Some causes of PIDs include chlamydia, cystitis, gonorrhea, various viruses, or anything that triggers the natural bacterial flora of the vagina to foster an infection, such as childbirth, reproductive system surgery, abortion, or use of an intrauterine device (IUD).

Natural remedies for PID include nutritional supplements (acidophilus, zinc, and vitamins C and E; see Chapter 4); herbs (aloe vera, astragalus, echinacea, garlic) and homeopathy (aconite, apis, colocynthis, graphites, lycopodium, and mercurius; see Chapter 5).

Prostatic and Testicular Conditions

The "male gland," or prostate gland, is a walnut-size organ situated just below the bladder and next to the rectum. The prostate gland wraps around the urethra. Thus when the gland becomes inflamed or enlarged, it restricts the flow of urine and causes pain. The testicles are two small organs located in the scrotum behind the penis. Because of their position and the fact that they are highly sensitive, they are susceptible to injury. Any swelling of the testicles should be addressed by a physician.

Prostate enlargement, or *benign prostatic hyperplasia,* occurs in approximately 50 to 60 percent of men ages 40 to 59 years. It can progress quickly or advance very slowly and stop. Researchers believe genetics and lifestyle (e.g., lack of exercise) have the most impact on the progression of the disease. Loss of libido is a common side effect.

Inflammation or infection of the prostate gland, called *prostatitis,* causes symptoms that are similar to those of benign prostatic hypertrophy: difficulty urinating, dribbling, blood in the urine, chills and fever, and aching in the area of the prostate. Loss of sexual desire is usually a temporary side effect.

Prostate cancer occurs in one of eight American men. Symptoms include an enlarged prostate that is hard to the touch. Other symptoms include an urge to urinate frequently, pain when urinating, and blood in the urine.

Problems that affect the testicles and threaten sexual fitness include *tortion of the testicles, orchitis, cancer, swelling,* and *undescended testicles.* Torsion of the testicles, which usually occurs during puberty, is the twisting of the testicles around themselves in the scrotum, which cuts off the blood flow. Immediate emergency medical care is needed to save the testicles and maintain fertility. If the damaged testicle needs to be removed surgically, the remaining testicle is sufficient for a man to remain fertile.

Orchitis is inflammation and infection of one or both testicles. This painful condition is often accompanied by fever. Orchitis may cause a man to become infertile.

Cases of testicular cancer are most commonly seen among men ages 20 to 35. It is the third leading cause of death among men ages 20 to 40. Signs include a firm, painless swelling in the testicle that may be accompanied by inflammation. The greatest risk factor for this type of cancer is an undescended testicle that is not corrected before the age of two.

Swelling of the testicles is usually harmless; however, if it is caused by a viral or bacterial infection, it may reduce a man's sperm count. About 10 to 15 percent of men experience a swelling condition known as *varicocele,* which is a clustering of varicose veins above the left testicle. This painful condition raises the temperature of the testicles and lowers the sperm count.

Among men who undergo prostate or testicular surgery, a condition known as "dry orgasm" occurs. These men do not ejaculate because they no longer produce sperm. Prostate surgery performed because of cancer results in impotence in 40 percent or more of men, depending on the type of surgery done. A type of surgery done for an enlarged prostate, or benign prostatic hyperplasia (BPH), rarely causes impotence, although about 90 percent of men who undergo the surgery (which is called *transurethral resection,* or TUR) experience retrograde ejaculation, in which the semen goes backward into the bladder with orgasm.

Natural remedies to help avoid prostate and testicular problems or to treat current ones include various foods and nutritional supplements (watercress leaves, sesame seeds, pumpkin seeds, lecithin, calcium, magnesium, evening primrose oil, cold-pressed linseed oil, flower pollen; see Chapter 4); herbal remedies (couchgrass, damiana, ginseng, horsetail, pygeum, saw palmetto) and homeopathic remedies (argentum nitricum, baryta carbonate, conium, lycopodium, pulsatilla; see Chapter 5). And while some people say clothing makes the man, men who want to help preserve their sexual health need to avoid wearing tight briefs and pants, as they restrict blood flow and raise the temperature of the scrotum, which reduces sperm count.

Sexually Transmitted Diseases

Whenever two people embark on a sexual relationship, the possibility that they will share more than intimate moments is all too real in today's society. The rate of infection of sexually transmitted diseases, or STDs, is on the rise. Sexual partners need to be open and honest with each other about the state of their health before they engage in sexual activity. Human immunodeficiency virus (HIV), gonorrhea, herpes, chlamydia, syphilis, and human papilloma virus are the most common of the more than 50 STDs.

In addition to the symptoms of these diseases, the psychological trauma that often accompanies the stigma of having any of them can undermine a relationship. It takes understanding and trust on the part of both partners to weather the treatment period and to rebuild from any emotional damage that has been done.

Human immunodeficiency virus (HIV) is a deadly disease in which individuals experience progressive damage to their immune system until the body is unable to defend itself against infection. Between 70 and 85 percent of cases are transmitted by penetrative sex. It is believed most of these cases could be prevented if people practiced safe sex. (See Chapter 1.) The remaining numbers are caused by needle sharing among drug users, blood transfusions, and infected pregnant women passing it along to their infants.

As many as 65 percent of people infected with HIV go on to develop AIDS—acquired immunodeficiency syndrome. The only way to make a positive diagnosis is to have a blood test. If you suspect you may have contracted HIV, you can be tested anonymously at a clinic that specializes in HIV/AIDS.

Acquired immunodeficiency syndrome has four stages. Stage 1 is the acute infection stage. Up to 25 percent of people have initial symptoms two to five weeks after they become infected with HIV. Symptoms include body aches, fever, chills, ulcers in the genital area, and sore throat. During stage 2, symptoms disappear, although some people get swelling of the lymph nodes in the neck, groin, and armpits. This stage can last up to ten years or longer. Symptoms return in stage 3 because the immune system reaches a critical point. Common symptoms include fatigue, diarrhea, weight loss, and high susceptibility to infection. By stage 4, the immune system breaks down further, allowing infections such as tuberculosis, encephalitis, pneumonia, or herpes to take control. In many cases death occurs within four years of a person entering stage 4. Various drug combinations are used to treat HIV/AIDS.

Gonorrhea is caused by the bacterium *Neisseria gonorrhoeae* and is transmitted during unprotected vaginal or anal sex and during oral sex. Many people with gonorrhea are symptom-free, especially women. Among men the symptoms are a discharge from the penis or anus and pain when defecating or urinating. Women may experience a yellow discharge from the vagina or urethra and a frequent need to urinate.

If untreated, gonorrhea in men can cause an infection of the prostate gland and possibly result in infertility. In women gonorrhea can cause pelvic inflammatory disease and fertility difficulties. Infants born to women with gonorrhea may develop serious illness or become blind. Conventional treatment of gonorrhea consists of antibiotics.

Chlamydia trachomatis is an organism that has characteristics of both bacteria and viruses. It causes an infection that can jeopardize both a man and woman's fertility. Approximately one-half million new cases are reported each year to the Centers for Disease Control and Prevention. Because doctors are not required to report chlamydia, the actual number may be as high as 3 to 10 million.

Chlamydia is difficult to detect in women because it usually does not cause any symptoms until it reaches the fallopian tubes and causes pelvic inflammatory disease. (See "Pelvic Inflammatory Disease," p. 56.) A Pap smear cannot detect chlamydia; you need to ask your physician to do a *Chlamydia* culture. Chlamydia is the most common and most serious male genitourinary tract infection. The symptoms include burning pain when urinating and a watery or yellow discharge from the urethra. Without prompt treatment, *Chlamydia* may cause infections of the prostate gland, rectum, and epididymis. Low sperm counts are attributed to chlamydia infection, and this disease is estimated to be associated with male infertility in up to 71 percent of cases. Standard treatment of chlamydia consists of antibiotics. Natural approaches include proper hydration, zinc supplementation (see Chapter 4) and herbal remedies, such as echinacea, which is explained in Chapter 5, and other herbs not covered here, such as uva ursi, goldenseal, and bromelain. (See Appendix B for information on herbs and herbal sources.)

Syphilis is a bacterial infection that is spread by vaginal or anal intercourse, oral sex, kissing, skin-to-skin contact, shared needles among drug abusers, and infected blood transfusions. If left untreated (antibiotics are standard therapy), it can be fatal.

Signs of syphilis initially include a lump that develops into a sore, or chancre. After the chancre disappears, the lymph nodes may enlarge and be accompanied by red spots on the hands, feet, and other body parts. Headache, low-grade fever, sore throat, and hair loss also may occur. The disease then enters a latent period during which the infected individual feels healthy. Those who are left untreated then enter the final stage, which includes brain damage, paralysis, and cardiovascular problems.

Human papilloma virus (*HPV*), also known as *genital warts,* is a serious STD and one of the most difficult to detect. According to King Holmes, M.D., at the University of Washington School of Medicine in Seattle, it is the most common STD in women, yet most of them don't know they have it. Approximately 80 percent of the population carries the virus, yet most do not develop symptoms. When they do, they include warts that appear on the cervix, urethra, rectum, vagina, and vulva. Some strains of the virus are associated with cancer of the cervix, vagina, penis, or vulva.

The best natural protection against the virus is to boost the immune system with supplements of zinc and folic acid and vitamins A, C, and E. An effective herbal remedy is Chuan Xin Lian Kang Yang Pian, which contains the herb isatis. It is available through Chinese herb stores. (See Appendix B.)

Herpes is a viral infection that is difficult to detect unless the sores are cultured during an acute stage. Both types of herpesvirus—herpes simplex 1 and herpes simplex 2—cause sores, although simplex 2 is the form responsible for the genital sores. Signs and symptoms include itching or tingling in the genital area, swollen and tender lymph nodes, low-grade fever, and general malaise. Men often experience painful blisters on the glans of the penis while women may have blisters in the vagina, cervix, or perineum. Women can pass the infection along to their infants during childbirth, and the children run the risk of brain infections and blindness.

There is no cure for herpes, although the frequency of attacks can be reduced with antiviral drugs and use of the amino acid L-lysine (up to 3,000 mg per day). It also helps to avoid foods that contain arginine, which stimulates the growth of the viruses. Arginine is found in seeds, nuts, wheat, and chocolate. Herbal remedies to help relieve symptoms and reduce herpes attacks include astragalus, suma, and ashwaganda. The Chinese formula Chuan Xin Lian Kang Yang Pian (available through Chinese herbalists, some traditional herbalists, and mail order), as well as supplements of zinc and vitamins A, C, and E are helpful.

Surgery

Several surgical procedures can have an impact on sexual fitness and functioning, particularly amputation of a limb, colostomy, hysterectomy, mastectomy, and prostatectomy. In all cases, psychological effects are commonly a factor, as individuals who have undergone any of these procedures may feel "less than" a complete man or woman or worry that no one will find them attractive anymore. Thus lack of self-esteem and confidence may be the biggest and only hurdle stopping them from enjoying sexual relations.

You have learned about the intricate relationship between overall health and sexual health. To enjoy sexual fitness, you need to gain and maintain the optimal overall fitness level possible for you. But enough about what can go wrong. Let's move on to how to improve your sexual fitness.

CHAPTER FOUR

Fueled for Sex: Food and Nutritional Supplements

Sexual fitness begins with the fuel you put into your body. The quality and quantity of food, beverages, and supplements you choose have a major impact on your sexual health, including your level of sexual desire; how much strength, stamina, and flexibility you will have for sexual activity; and how well you will be able to maintain a healthy weight.

Many nutrition experts and medical organizations have established nutritional guidelines to help people move toward and maintain both overall health and sexual fitness. In this chapter you can learn what types of foods and supplements health professionals suggest for sexual fitness and how to incorporate their suggestions into your daily eating plan.

Basic Food-for-Sexual-Fitness Plan

In recent years medical experts have been gathering an enormous amount of evidence about the benefits of a low-fat, low-cholesterol, and higher fiber and carbohydrate eating plan that consists of whole, natural foods. This approach can provide most people with the energy, stamina, and overall vitality they need for sexual fitness. It also promotes a healthy reproductive system and helps prevent diseases that can hinder sexual activity, such as cancer, high blood pressure, obesity, and diabetes. According to James F. Balch and Phyllis Balch, authors of *Prescription for Nutritional Healing,* diet is one of the most important factors in maintaining sexual fitness, and vitamin supplements have a critical role in increasing and maintaining sexual energy.

Although many Americans say they want to eat healthier foods, often they think it's too much trouble to prepare something that's "good for them" or they think healthful food is "boring." One of the biggest hurdles, however, is that they like the foods they eat now and don't really want to change. Change can be uncomfortable, inconvenient, and scary. But it need not be any of those things. And when the result is more sexual energy and vitality and better overall health, change can be something to look forward to!

The following text outlines the basics of a food plan for sexual fitness. See how your current diet stacks up and then get ready for some positive and tasty changes.

Endless Energy: Complex Carbohydrates

Carbohydrates are one of the three main types of food and the one that should make up 60 to 65 percent of the food you eat. Protein and fats, the other two types of foods, are explained elsewhere in this chapter.

Simple and Complex. Carbohydrates come in two forms: simple and complex. Simple carbohydrates include sugar in all its forms, including white and brown sugars, honey, sodas, and candy. These foods burn rapidly in the body and so provide a quick burst of energy followed by an energy lull. Complex carbohydrates help keep your energy level even because they burn slowly. Whole grains and products made from them, such as breads, pasta, and cereals, as well as rice, sprouts, legumes, beans, vegetables, and soybean products, provide complex carbohydrates. These are energy foods, which are needed for sexual stamina and endurance. Many of these foods are also good sources of protein.

Sexy Carbohydrates. Include complex carbohydrates at every meal to keep your sexual energy and fitness level up. Here are some ideas:

- Breakfast: oatmeal with soy milk; whole-grain toast, muffin, or bagel with naturally sweetened jam; homefries (use spray-on oil) with sautéed mushrooms, peppers, and tomatoes; whole-grain cereal with fruit; bean burrito with salsa; scrambled tofu with tomatoes, peppers, and mushrooms; potato pancakes; granola with soy milk

- Lunch and Dinner: lentil soup; black bean or navy bean soup; stir-fried brown rice and vegetables; wheat pita stuffed with bean spread and sprouts; soy burger on wheat roll; bean chili; corn chowder; wheat macaroni salad with chopped fresh vegetables; spinach salad with croutons and garbanzo beans; vegetable lasagna

Tens of thousands of healthful recipes, many of them fast and easy, can be found in cookbooks, magazines, and on the Internet. (See Suggested Readings for a sample of what's available in bookstores, libraries, and online.)

The Protein Push

A phenomenon called the "Protein Myth" has been circulating throughout the United States for many years. Americans worry about getting enough protein, when in fact people in this country typically consume too much protein, especially in the form of meat and dairy products, which usually are also high in fat and cholesterol. (See the box "How Much Protein Do I Need?, p. 71.)

Beware of high-protein diets, such as the Atkins Diet and the Zone. Groups such as the American Dietetic Association, The American College of Sports Medicine, the Cooper Institute for Aerobics Research, and the Women's Sports Foundation, and many other experts point out that excess protein weakens the prostate, kidneys, and bladder. This, in turn, is detrimental to sexual fitness. It is also harder for the body to burn off excess protein than it is to burn carbohydrates and fats. People who consume a high-protein diet typically feel fatigued, which limits their sexual fitness and interest in sex.

Plant- vs. Animal-based Proteins. Plant-based proteins can be easily substituted for animal-derived sources, and by doing so you leave behind most of the fat and all of the cholesterol. It is not necessary to combine certain plant proteins at the same meal. As long as you eat a variety of healthful foods, your body knows how to make complete proteins from incomplete ones. In fact, many plant proteins go together naturally to make complete protein meals.

Sexy Proteins. Consider these tasty combinations:

- Whole-wheat pasta and tomato sauce
- Falafel on wheat pita
- Beans and rice
- Whole-grain cereal and rice or soy milk
- Peanut butter on whole-grain bread
- Lentil soup with pasta
- Stir-fried tofu and vegetables with brown rice
- Baked potato stuffed with broccoli and white sauce
- Bean tortillas

You'll notice that many foods in the complex carbohydrate category also fall into the plant-based protein category. That's because these foods are great sources of each!

HOW MUCH PROTEIN DO I NEED?

It's easy to compute: Simply multiply your *ideal* weight (not how much you actually weigh, but what you should weigh based on your height, age, and bone structure) by 0.36 if you are 19 years or older. Thus, if you are a 30-year-old man who does (or should) weigh 170 pounds, you need 0.36 × 170 = 61.2 grams of protein per day. A 50-year-old, 120-pound woman needs 43 grams per day. These figures are similar to those recommended by the World Health Organization (WHO). Yet many Americans eat 90 grams or more per day.

Fat

Fat is another often misunderstood element in the diet. One reason for the confusion is that there are several types of fat—some healthy and some not. Another source of misunderstanding is the misconception that all fat is bad. In fact, fat is a critical part of the diet. Your brain is largely composed of fat, and fat is needed to conduct many of the body's functions.

Americans eat too much fat, and the excess robs the body of energy, including sexual energy, and its ability to fight disease. That's because most fats become rancid when they encounter oxygen, and then they turn into cell-destroying, disease-causing elements called free radicals.

Fat Squashes Sexual Desire. Fat cells contain a lot of aromatase, which is an enzyme that converts testosterone to estrogen. The more fat and fat cells you have in your body, the higher your estrogen levels can be. High estrogen levels in relation to testosterone can place a damper on sexual desire in men.

Fat Slows the Flow. Your body needs some fat to function optimally, so it's best to eat those foods that contain healthful fats. All foods contain some fat: Even apples and carrots have a minute amount. But *saturated fats* are one of the types of fat to avoid. These are found in meat, cheese, milk and other dairy products, poultry, and tropical oils. Saturated fats raise the "bad" cholesterol levels (known as LDL, or low-density lipoprotein cholesterol) in the blood. High LDL levels cause blood flow to become sluggish, which is a problem among men who are impotent. High cholesterol levels also cause an imbalance in sex hormone levels and increase the risk of prostate and breast cancers, heart attack, stroke, and arthritis.

Other Fats That Hamper Sexual Fitness. The most common fat in today's processed foods is polyunsaturated fat. This fat is found in prepackaged items such as cereals, crackers, cookies, dinner mixes, chips, frostings, condiments and sauces, salad dressings, puddings, peanut butter, and frozen foods. Polyunsaturated fats raise the level of triglycerides (fats in the blood).

Most margarines and many processed foods also contain *hydrogenated and partially hydrogenated fats*. These fats are manufactured by adding hydrogen to vegetable oil to create a solid, saturated fat. The result is a type of fat that has a high percentage of trans fatty acids, which the body cannot process effectively. A trans fatty acid is a manmade fat that is created when liquid fats such as corn oil are changed into hydrogenated or partially hydrogenated fats. As the body tries to rid itself of trans fatty acids, the process can cause problems, such as an increased risk of prostate and breast cancers and heart disease.

Sexy Fats. Healthful fats are found in vegetable and nut oils, including olive, canola, macadamia, and flaxseed, as well as in nuts, seeds, and avocados. According to Andrew Weil, M.D., a pioneer in complementary medicine and author of many books, including *Natural Health, Natural Medicine,* substituting these "good" fats for the "bad" ones such as palm and coconut oils, mayonnaise, and whole milk, is a wise choice. Healthful fats, in moderation, do not increase the risk of heart disease or become carcinogenic, and they also help lower the levels of bad cholesterol. All of these benefits mean a healthier heart, better blood circulation, and more sexual energy.

How Much Fat Do I Need? The American Dietetic Association and American Heart Association recommend that less than 30 percent of your total caloric intake consists of fat. Between 15 and 25 percent is preferred, especially if you need to lose weight or have a condition such as breast cancer, hypertension, diabetes, or heart disease. If your recommended caloric intake is 2,000 per day, 300 to 500 calories should come from fat. In fat grams, that's 33 to 55 grams of fat per day. (Divide 300 and 500 by 9, which is the number of calories per gram of fat.)

A Link Between Fat and Estrogen. The major cause of hormonal imbalance in women—high estrogen levels—is too much dietary fat. Fat cells not only store fat, they also produce estrogen. The more fat you eat, the more estrogen your body produces. In addition, a diet that contains too much fat, animal protein, and refined foods causes the body to keep recirculating estrogen through the body, which can cause the body to produce substances that can lead to hormone-related cancers, such as cancer of the uterus, breast, and ovaries. High saturated fat also prevents the liver from breaking down female hormones and thus promotes production of hormones that cause menstrual cramps and mood swings.

Sugar and Sex: How Sweet It's Not

Sex can be sweet, but you don't need the sugar. The average American eats between 30 and 40 teaspoons of sugar per day, much of it hidden in processed foods and beverages. According to Julian Whitaker, M.D., author of *Dr. Whitaker's Guide to Natural Health*, *Reversing Diabetes*, and *Reversing Health Risks*, the food industry is placing the health of Americans in jeopardy because of the amount of sugar it adds to food. Excess sugar opens the door to many medical problems that affect both sexual fitness and overall health, including chronic fatigue, candidiasis, calcium deficiency and bone loss, and depletion of minerals, B vitamins, and vitamin C in the body.

The Sexy Soybean

Soybeans and products made from them, which include tofu, tempeh, tamari, miso, and soy sauce, offer many health benefits, not least of which is the ability to fight cancer. In the sexual arena, soy products are valued because they contain isoflavones, a type of phytoestrogen. Once in the body, phytoestrogens prevent some of the activities of the body's natural estrogen from occurring, thus decreasing estrogen's libido-lowering effects in men.

Women also can enjoy better sexual fitness from eating soy foods. For many women, the phytoestrogens in soy products stabilize their estrogen levels and relieve symptoms of premenstrual syndrome (PMS). Soybeans also provide high levels of essential fatty acids, protein, calcium, potassium, vitamin C, and other nutrients.

Eat Your Veggies

Besides being a wonderful source of vitamins, minerals, fiber, and carbohydrates, some vegetables can help with sexual fitness. The cruciferous vegetables, such as cauliflower, broccoli, kale, radishes, bok choy, brussels sprouts, arugula, cabbage, and watercress, help the body burn off extra estrogen. In men, excess estrogen in relation to testosterone can cause loss of sexual desire. (See Chapter 3.)

Fiber Fitness

Fiber is a substance found in plant-based foods that helps eliminate toxins and cholesterol from the body through the feces. Fiber comes in two forms: water soluble and insoluble. Most foods that contain fiber have both types, although one kind usually dominates. Water-soluble fiber helps reduce blood cholesterol, and insoluble fiber helps normalize bowel function and move poisons out of the body more rapidly. But fiber also has another function that is related to sexual fitness.

Dietary fiber has the task of reducing the amount of estrogens in the body. Several studies have shown that women who eat a plant-based diet eliminate two to three times more estrogen in their feces than women who are not vegetarians. Excess estrogen in women is associated with breast, ovarian, and uterine cancers, dysmenorrhea, fibroids of the uterus, fibrocystic breast disease, and problems with menopause. In men, too much estrogen can cause a loss of sexual desire. (See Chapter 3.)

Most health care practitioners recommend a daily fiber intake of 20 to 35 grams, yet Americans typically consume about 11. It's easy to see why: Meat, fowl, fish, and dairy products, which make up a large part of the American diet, do not contain fiber. Substituting plant-based foods such as beans, whole grains and cereals, legumes, seeds, vegetables, fruits, and nuts for animal-derived foods will immediately increase your fiber intake.

Summary of Food for Sexual Fitness

For maximum sexual fitness and overall health, follow the guidelines explained in the box on pages 79–80. Most of these dietary recommendations were provided by the Diet & Cancer Project, an intensive research effort conducted by the American Institute for Cancer Research and the World Cancer Research Foundation. The findings result from a review of more than 4,500 studies of diet and cancer and explain how to build a balanced diet for overall good health and cancer and disease prevention. The recommendations apply especially to sexual health, as both breast and prostate cancers are two of the most prevalent cancers affecting people today.

Chinese Medicine Diet for Sexual Fitness

According to Chinese medicine, the kidneys are the source of sexual vitality, and the flow of energy from the kidneys (called kidney yang) to the sex organs sparks sexual desire. Thus the kidneys need to be healthy and well nourished to support sexual fitness in general in both men and women and to treat impotence in particular. Chinese medicine teaches that the spleen, heart, and circulatory system must be treated to maintain kidney yang.

The Chinese recommend the following dietary guidelines to strengthen kidney yang and to help cure impotence.

- Eat these foods often: whole grains (especially brown rice, oats, and sweet rice), high-carbohydrate vegetables (carrots, turnips, winter squash, sweet potatoes, yams, and pumpkin), and pungent foods such as onions, leeks, ginger, garlic, fennel, and black pepper.
- These foods are especially good for strengthening kidney yang: fenugreek seeds, anise seeds, cinnamon, walnuts, black beans, quinoa (a grain high in protein), salmon.
- These foods help resolve impotence: green vegetables, seeds (especially pumpkin and sunflower), wheat germ, seaweed, sprouted beans and seeds.
- Eat these foods rarely or avoid if you are impotent: fruits, tomatoes, spinach, tofu, vinegar, cold foods and drinks, salty foods, excessive raw vegetables.
- Avoid these foods completely: meat, eggs, dairy

Summary of Dietary Recommendations

For General Sexual Health

- Select whole, natural, unprocessed foods whenever possible.
- Select a diet that is primarily plant-based. This includes vegetables, fruits, grains, pasta, breads, rice, legumes and beans, seeds, nuts, and sea vegetables.
- Eat at least five servings of fruits and vegetables every day.
- Eliminate red meat. If you choose to eat it, limit consumption to less than 3 ounces per day.
- Eliminate animal protein. If it is eaten, limit consumption to a few ounces of fish or chicken, without skin, and prepared without fat.
- Eat at least seven servings of grains, legumes, roots, tubers, and plantains per day.
- Limit consumption of fatty foods, including fried foods, dairy and other animal products, and oils. Use vegetable oils in moderation.
- Avoid or limit alcohol consumption. For women, limit to one drink per day; for men, two.
- Avoid eating food that has been charred or burned. Such foods typically contain high amounts of cancer-causing substances.
- Replace the salt shaker with herbs and spices. Avoid salty foods.
- Drink eight glasses of pure water daily.
- Store perishable foods properly.
- Avoid sugar and caffeine.

For Specific Sexual-Fitness Concerns

- For impotence, include foods rich in zinc: 1/2 cup pumpkin seeds per day is recommended; also add sesame seeds and avocados to your diet. (Also see "Zinc," under "Sexy Supplements.")
- For prostate problems, avoid coffee (caffeinated and decaffeinated) and red pepper Include sesame and pumpkin seeds, cold-pressed linseed oil, and watercress leaves.
- For dysmenorrhea, include beets and foods rich in vitamin B6. (See "B Vitamins," under "Sexy Supplements.")
- For infertility, eat foods rich in essential fatty acids, zinc, vitamins E and B6. (See individual nutrients listed under "Sexy Supplements.")
- For loss of sex drive, painful periods, and menopause, include soy products (tofu, tempeh, miso, soy milk, soy cheese, soy burgers, and soy yogurt) and cruciferous vegetables (broccoli, cauliflower, bok choy, radishes, cabbage, brussels sprouts).
- For premature ejaculation, avoid caffeine.

products, sugar, poultry, alcohol, any high-fat foods.

Sexy Supplements

First and foremost, to ensure sexual fitness, provide your body with the freshest and most nutritious food and drink possible, as was discussed earlier. No matter how wholesome you believe food to be, many factors can have a detrimental effect on how the body processes the food you eat. Emotional and physical stress, the fact that many foods lack a sufficient amount of vital nutrients, the presence of chemical additives in many foods, and the harmful effects of environmental pollutants all take a toll on your health and sexual fitness.

Supplements are like insurance policies. Not only do they allow you to help ward off nutritional deficiencies and medical problems by taking a tablet, capsule, powder, or liquid one or more times a day, they also can improve the quality of your sexual fitness by giving you more energy and stamina and helping you resolve sexual difficulties such as impotence and low sexual desire.

A brief explanation of some of the specific vitamins, minerals, and other nutrients that can boost your sexual health and fitness follows. Although the body needs many different nutrients to function at its best, taking more than the recommended amount of any supplement can upset the balance of other nutrients in the body. Therefore, talk with your physician before you begin a supplement program. Table 4.1, a chart of the supplements that can help ensure optimal general health (which includes sexual health), is provided at the end of this chapter.

Acidophilus

Acidophilus is a form of bacteria, *Lactobacillus acidophilus,* that can help protect against and treat yeast infections (including candidiasis and moniliasis) and urinary tract infections. Yeast infections can cause painful sexual intercourse as well as fatigue and a loss of interest in sex. Acidophilus can restore a healthy bacterial environment to the vagina and intestines. Along with taking supplements of acidophilus, women with a yeast infection should avoid using tampons and douches (unless using an acidophilus douche, as described below), eliminate sugar from the diet, and stop taking birth control pills and antibiotics.

How to Take/Food Sources. Acidophilus is available as a powdered supplement and in foods, such as acidophilus milk and some yogurts. (Buy yogurt that contains *Lactobacillus* [or *L.*] *acidophilus.*) Nondairy varieties of acidophilus, which use carrot juice as their base, are also available. If you experience frequent yeast infections or if you occasionally take antibiotics, add acidophilus to your diet to help maintain a healthy vagina and intestinal tract.

Another way to restore the healthy bacteria to the vagina is to use an acidophilus douche twice a day. Dissolve 10 milliliters (ml) of an acidophilus supplement or an active-culture yogurt in 10 ml of water. Use a syringe to douche the solution into the vagina. Hold the solution as long as is comfortable, then release. This type of douche is usually safe and nonirritating.

B Vitamins

The B vitamin family works synergistically; therefore, it should be taken as a B-complex supplement. The complex is especially helpful in relieving menopausal symptoms. Supplementation with B6 is recommended for men and women who are experiencing infertility and for women with dysmenorrhea, who also need B12.

Excessive estrogen levels are associated with a deficiency of the B vitamins, especially vitamins B6 and B12. The liver, which breaks down and inactivates estrogen in the body, needs B vitamins to do its job.

How to Take. Individuals who are experiencing infertility and/or dysmenorrhea can take a B complex plus additional vitamin B6 (50 to 300 milligrams [mg] daily) and B12 (200 to 1,000 micrograms [mcg]). For menopause, a vitamin B-complex supplement that contains 50 to 100 mg of the B vitamins is recommended. (See Table 4.1.)

Food Sources. Vitamin B complex: whole grains and legumes; Vitamin B6: brewer's yeast, broccoli, brown rice, brussels sprouts, green peas, soybeans, rice bran, lentils, lima beans, pinto beans, asparagus, sweet potatoes. Vitamin B12: brewer's yeast, cereals fortified with B12; sea vegetables, such as dulse nori, kombu, and kelp; herbs such as alfalfa, hops, and bladderwrack; and soybeans and soy products such as miso and tempeh. Nonvegetable sources include liver, clams, herring, mackerel, dairy products, and eggs.

Note. Vitamin B6 can be toxic if you take more than 500 mg daily for many months or years. Symptoms include tingling sensations in the feet, degeneration of nerve tissue, and loss of muscle coordination. Absorption of B12 can be hindered if you take anticoagulants, antigout drugs, or potassium supplements.

Bee Pollen and Pollen Extract

Bee pollen is one of nature's most nutritious and most mysterious substances. After bees gather pollen, they add as-yet-unidentified ingredients to it. The result is a product that stimulates human sex glands and hormone production, which results in an increase in sexual potency. Bee pollen also boosts the immune system, reduces fatigue, and helps heal cuts and burns. Since ancient times, this "ambrosia of the gods" has been revered for its ability to promote perpetual youth and health.

One reason bee pollen has these abilities is because it is nutrient rich: It contains 22 amino acids, including all the essential ones; 27 minerals, including calcium, iron, and magnesium; enzymes; and all vitamins, including B12.

Another pollen product is pollen extract, which is pollen gathered from plants and then extracted in a laboratory. Although bee pollen has been used medicinally for centuries, pollen extracts are just beginning to be appreciated for their ability to heal. Pollen extracts provide several physical advantages, including smooth muscle relaxation and anti-inflammatory action, both of which are important to sexual fitness.

For men with prostate problems, it is important that the smooth muscles in the bladder relax. When the muscles at the neck of the bladder are tense and spasms occur, urinary problems can result. These problems are often accompanied by prostatitis. Pollen extract causes the bladder muscles to relax and allows urine to be eliminated. The anti-inflammatory action of pollen extract is key in the treatment of an enlarged or inflamed prostate gland.

Some researchers believe pollen extract is superior to saw palmetto, another herb that is effective in treating prostate problems, although both provide good results. (See "Saw Palmetto," p. 120.) According to Dallas Clouatre, Ph.D., author of *Pollen Extract for Prostate Health,* "Saw palmetto does have an established track record with prostate problems. Unfortunately, it typically takes a very long time to work, about two or three months minimum, and you have to take quite a bit. It's not that saw palmetto is bad, I think the flower pollen extracts are better."

How to Take. Bee pollen is available in capsules and can be taken either as a supplement or mixed with food, such as soups, puddings, and rice. Take according to package directions. Pollen extract usually comes in tablets with instructions to take one to two twice a day with meals. Follow package directions.

Note. If you add bee pollen to food, do so after the

food has been cooked, because heating bee pollen destroys its nutritional value.

Calcium

Calcium is often thought of as a woman's supplement to help prevent osteoporosis, and indeed it plays this important role. Yet men also need to pay attention to this mineral. Calcium plays a critical part in nerve transmission. Thus men who want to help maintain prostatic and testicular health are encouraged to get an adequate amount of calcium. The current Recommended Daily Allowance (RDA) of calcium for adults is 800–1,500 mg per day.

Calcium also is involved in muscle contractions, which are so important in orgasm. Very low levels of calcium in the blood can contribute to muscle spasms and leg cramps, which can hinder sexual activity if they strike in the heat of passion.

How to Take. Andrew Weil, M.D., recommends taking 1,000 to 1,500 mg per day, with two-thirds at bedtime and one-third in the morning. Calcium should always be taken along with magnesium, because a proper balance of the two is required for transmission of signals to the nerves and muscles. Dr. Weil recommends a 1:1 ratio. (If you take 1,000 mg calcium, take 1,000 mg magnesium.) Some physicians suggest a 2:1 ratio of calcium to magnesium. In either case look for supplements that combine the two minerals.

Food Sources. Greens, such as collards, kale, mustard; broccoli, tofu, fortified orange juice, sesame seeds, molasses. Dairy sources are not recommended as they speed up the loss of calcium from bones.

Note. Calcium citrate is the best-absorbed calcium supplement. Calcium carbonate is a good alternative. Avoid calcium supplements that consist of natural oyster shell, dolomite, and bone meal, as they typically contain lead. Foods and products that increase the amount of calcium excreted from the body include caffeine, alcohol, protein, salt, sugar, and aluminum-containing antacids. Avoid these products as much as possible and limit your protein intake to no more than 20 percent of your caloric intake to get the most benefit from your calcium supplement.

DHEA

DHEA (dehydroepiadrosterone) is an androgen (male hormone) and the most abundant hormone in the human bloodstream. It is produced by the adrenal gland and works synergistically with at least 18 other hormones in the body, including the sex hormones testosterone, estrogen, and progesterone.

Many people use DHEA to help improve sex drive and stamina. It has been the subject of more than 10,000 scientific papers and numerous studies, and thus far many of the findings support these claims. In July 1995 researchers at a scientific meeting in Washington, D.C., run under the auspices of The New York Academy of Sciences, announced that DHEA improved libido (with dramatic results in women) as well as increased energy and cognitive function, enhanced the immune system, and allowed for more restful sleep. DHEA's effect on libido occurs when the hormone is converted into androgens and estrogens when it enters the bloodstream and the cells.

How to Take. Many medical researchers and physicians recommend taking supplements of DHEA after age 30, as the body's production of the hormone begins to decline when people are in their 20s. Note, however, that DHEA is a hormone and should be treated as a potent medication. DHEA should not be taken by anyone who has a personal or family history of tumors that respond to hormones, such as breast or prostate cancer. DHEA can cause acne, facial hair growth in women, fatigue, insomnia, irritability, and oily skin in some people.

The suggested dose is 25 mg daily for women and 50 mg daily for men. DHEA can be purchased over the counter and is available as a synthetic or an animal-derived extract. No natural alternative has yet been found. DHEA should be taken only in consultation with your medical practitioner.

Note: A substance derived from wild yams called *diosgenin* is sold as a precursor (a substance from which another product is formed) to DHEA. However, although it is possible to transform wild yam into DHEA in a laboratory, the body cannot do the same, and so wild yam does not actually function as a natural precursor to DHEA in the human body.

Essential Fatty Acids

Essential fatty acids consist of two fats—omega-3 and omega-6, also known as alpha-linolenic and alpha-linoleic, respectively—which the body needs to operate at its best. They are called "essential" because the body cannot manufacture them; they must be obtained through the diet.

Essential fatty acids (EFAs) promote sexual fitness because they are the precursors of prostaglandins, hormonelike substances that are involved in sexual response. Improving your sexual fitness may be as easy as supplementing your diet with EFAs, especially if you are among the more than 75 percent of Americans who are deficient in these nutrients. Essential fatty acids also are recommended to help prevent cancer and heart disease, to lower cholesterol levels, and to treat arthritis.

How to Take/Food Sources. Omega-3 oils are found in fish oils, especially cold-water fish, and in hemp seed oil. When looking for a supplement, you may see the words "eicosapentaenoic acid (EPA)" and "docosahexaenoic acid (DHA)," two common types of omega-3 supplements. Of the omega-6 oils, the most widely used supplement is gamma-linolenic acid, or GLA. Gamma-linolenic acid is found in plant oils, such as evening primrose, borage, flaxseed, hemp seed, black currant, and rape seed.

To help prostaglandins metabolize most effectively, which in turn benefits sexual response, choose an EFA supplement that provides 150 to 350 mg GLA. Experts recommend a supplement that contains a ratio of four to six parts of omega-6 to one part omega-3. The ratio should appear on the label.

Most EFA supplements are available as both capsules and liquid. Flaxseed oil, which can be used to make salad dressings, is an excellent source of EFAs: Two tablespoons per day fulfill all your daily needs. Nuts and seeds are also good sources of EFAs.

Note. Evening primrose oil is a very rich source of GLA, which makes it effective in the metabolism of prostaglandins, some of which in turn help regulate the menstrual cycle, alleviate anxiety, and lower high blood pressure, among other benefits. Women who have breast cancer or a family history of breast cancer, however, should avoid taking evening primrose oil, as it promotes the production of estrogen, and breast cancer is hormone-driven. Black currant seed oil is a safe substitute. Evening primrose oil is considered safe for women without breast cancer issues.

Histidine

During orgasm, the skin flush that occurs is the work of histidine, an amino acid that, with a little help from vitamin C, transforms into histamine. Some men and women know histamines are active because they experience a stuffy nose or a change in their sinuses at the moment of orgasm.

The release of histamines is necessary for sexual arousal. Researchers at the Institute of Pharmacology and Experimental Therapy in Torino, Italy, conducted studies which indicate that a stable balance of histidine and histamine is essential to ensure the ability to reach orgasm for both men and women. People with low levels of histidine may improve their ability to experience sexual excitement and orgasm by taking a histidine supplement.

How to Take. Combine 50 mg histidine per day (not to exceed 150 mg per day) with vitamin B6 to increase the ability to experience sexual arousal and orgasm.

Note. Take on an empty stomach for best results.

Lecithin

Lecithin is a fatty acid found in large amounts in semen, in the gonads of both women and men, and in the pituitary and pineal glands. This has led some researchers to believe that lecithin supplements may increase sexual potency and prevent impotence.

How to Take. Lecithin supplements are available as granules, powder, liquid, and in oil-filled capsules. The recommended dose is up to 1 gram daily. If you choose the granules, take 2 tablespoons per day in the evening with juice. (Also see "Phosphorus," p. 94.)

Food Sources. Green leafy vegetables, soy products, oatmeal, grains, seeds, yeast, chocolate, seaweed, wheat germ, and peanuts.

Note. Lecithin supplements have a high fat content and tend to become rancid. Therefore, some practitioners suggest increasing intake of lecithin-rich foods rather than taking a supplement.

Magnesium

Magnesium, along with calcium, is important in nerve transmission and so helps maintain prostatic and testicular health. (See "Calcium," p. 86.) It also is used to treat symptoms associated with dysmenorrhea.

How to Take. Magnesium should be taken with calcium in a combination supplement. Some physicians recommend taking calcium and magnesium in a 2:1 ratio; others suggest a 1:1 supplement. Michael Murray, N.D., author of *Encyclopedia of Natural Medicine* and *Encyclopedia of Nutritional Supplements,* recommends 12 mg per 2.2 pounds body weight for people with prostate conditions or dysmenorrhea, which translates into 600 mg for a 110-pound person and 1,080 mg for a 200-pound person.

Food Sources. Tofu, legumes, whole grains, green leafy vegetables, seeds, and nuts.

Note. Do not take magnesium supplements if you have kidney disease or severe heart disease.

Phenylalanine and Tyrosine

These two substances have a special relationship in the body: Tyrosine, a nonessential amino acid, is produced from L-7 phenylalanine, an essential amino acid. Together they play a primary role in enhancing sexual arousal and sexual desire.

The letter "L" affixed to the word "phenylalanine" identifies it as one of three forms of the amino acid. (D- and DL-phenylalanine are the other two.) The L-phenylalanine form is the one that most aids in sexual functioning because it is responsible for forming three substances important in sexual arousal—dopamine, norepinephrine, and epinephrine. An adequate amount of L-phenylalanine is also necessary to maintain the body's level of the neuropeptide phenyethylamine, a substance that is often absent in men and women who have little or no sex drive. People who lack tyrosine experience a deficiency of norepinephrine in the brain, which results in depression.

How to Take. Both amino acids should be taken when you first get up in the morning and at least 20 to 30 minutes before eating. This approach helps prevent other amino acids in foods from hindering absorption of the supplements. The average dose of L-phenylalanine is 375 to 500 mg; of tyrosine, 500 mg. The effectiveness of one or both amino acids is improved by taking 25 to 50 mg vitamin B6 plus 250 to 500 mg vitamin C at the same time.

Note. Neither amino acid should be taken by anyone who has malignant melanomas or who is pregnant, lactating, taking monoamine oxidase inhibitors (MAOIs), or who has psychosis. L-phenylalanine should not be taken by individuals who have high blood pressure.

Phosphorus

Phosphorus plays an integral part in helping the pancreas, thyroid, and adrenal glands produce sex hormones. If you are experiencing chronic stress, production of these hormones can decline dramatically, and with it your sexual desire and vitality.

How to Take. The RDA is 800 to 1,200 mg. When taking phosphorus supplements, make sure you take twice as much calcium as phosphorus (2:1 ratio), because calcium is necessary for phosphorus to function properly.

Food Sources. You can increase the amount of phosphorus in your diet easily by sprinkling wheat bran or wheat germ on your cereal or adding it to casseroles and by eating pumpkin and sunflower seeds. You can get an adequate supply of phosphorus if you take 2 tablespoons lecithin granules every evening in juice, along with 500 mg of vitamin E and 50 mg of vitamin B6.

Note. Too much magnesium can hinder the activity of phosphorus.

Selenium

Selenium promotes sperm production and assists in the functioning of the prostate gland.

How to Take. Take 50 to 100 mcg daily, depending on need.

Food Sources. Wheat germ, brazil nuts, oats, whole-wheat bread, red Swiss chard, bran, garlic, brown rice.

Note. Do not take more than 100 mcg per day. Take selenium at least 30 minutes after taking vitamin C supplements because they hinder each other's absorption.

Vitamin A

Vitamin A comes in two forms: carotene, which the body converts into vitamin A; and retinol, which enters the body already converted in the animals and animal products humans eat. Nutritionists consider beta-carotene, one of many carotenes, to be the better source of vitamin A.

Vitamin A is necessary for the production of the hormone progesterone and the production of sperm. When vitamin A and vitamin E are taken together, they can help increase a low sperm count. Low levels of vitamin A also have been linked to impotency.

How to Take. The suggested supplement dosage is 5,000 to 25,000 International Units (IU) for beta-carotene and 5,000 IU for retinol.

Food Sources. Spirulina, carrots, pumpkins, squash, sweet potatoes, yams, tomatoes, red peppers, dark green vegetables, and cantaloupe, apricots, and sour cherries.

Note. Supplementation of retinol up to 50,000 IU per day is safe. However, most experts recommend beta-carotene.

Vitamin C

Vitamin C (also known as ascorbic acid) is well known for its ability to fight off colds and flu, but it's also essential for healthy sperm and to treat infertility. Studies reported in the *Journal of the American Medical Association* and performed at the University of Texas Medical Branch in Galveston have shown that among men who have low levels of vitamin C and who are infertile because of sperm agglutination (clumping together), virility is restored once the body's vitamin C level is increased. That's because vitamin C protects the sperm's genetic material from damage. Researchers in several studies found virility was restored in men who took 1,000 to 3,000 mg vitamin C per day for 60 days.

How to Take. The RDA of vitamin C is only 60 mg, but most health care practitioners recommend 500 mg or more per day. If you smoke or regularly drink alcohol; or if you take birth control pills, estrogen, cortisone, or aspirin, 1,000 to 2,000 mg vitamin C is recommended, as tolerated.

Food Sources. Most vegetables and fruits, especially citrus, green peppers, cabbage, broccoli, cauliflower, and cantaloupe.

Note. Vitamin C is well tolerated by most people, although high doses may cause diarrhea in some individuals. This symptom is easily eliminated by reducing the dosage of vitamin C to a level that no longer causes the diarrhea.

Vitamin E

Vitamin E is a family of vitamins called tocopherols, which consists of alpha-, beta-, and gamma-tocopherol. Supplementation with vitamin E can help with infertility, painful intercourse, and various pelvic inflammatory diseases. Vitamin E has many roles in the body, including helping to maintain the immune system and the structure of the smooth muscles and to protect against fibrocystic breast disease.

How to Take. Supplementation is nearly always recommended because it is difficult to get your RDA of vitamin E solely from food. Take 400 to 600 IU per day; up to 1,200 if needed.

Food Sources. Broccoli, asparagus, whole grains, wheat germ, turnip greens, sweet potatoes, olive oil, safflower oil, and eggs.

Zinc

Zinc is perhaps the most important nutrient for good sexual health and fitness for both men and women. It is found in nearly every tissue and is part of more enzymatic processes than any other mineral in the human body. Yet most Americans do not get enough of this nutrient, and so it is also one of the most common ones lacking in the American diet.

A marginal zinc deficiency is enough to cause problems with sexual functioning. In men, an adequate level of zinc is critical for healthy sex hormone and prostate functioning. Low levels of zinc are associated with male infertility (a low sperm count) and a high rate of prostate enlargement. Women who experience pelvic inflammatory disease or menopause can benefit from zinc supplementation because it is a powerful immune system booster.

How to Take. The RDA for males 11 years and older is 15 mg; for females of the same age it is 12 mg, although pregnant and lactating women need up to 19 mg. The forms that are best absorbed are zinc picolinate, zinc citrate, and zinc momomethionine. Supplementation of 45 to 60 mg daily is recommended for men who are experiencing impotency or benign prostatic hyperplasia. A daily dose of 30 to 45 mg is recommended for women with pelvic inflammatory disease or who are going through menopause.

The body makes best use of zinc when there is an adequate supply of copper in the diet. You need only 2 to 3 mg copper per day to fulfill that need. Because zinc competes with other minerals for absorption, take your zinc supplement at least several hours before or after eating high-fiber foods and taking supplements of calcium and iron.

Food Sources. Pumpkin and sesame seeds are especially rich sources; other sources include sea vegetables, whole-grain foods, wheat germ, oysters, and soybeans. One ounce of wheat germ supplies 5 mg zinc, while two ounces of dried, hulled pumpkin seeds provides 4.2 mg.

Note. Zinc is nontoxic when taken as directed. A

dosage of 100 mg or more per day causes impaired immunity. At levels of 2 grams or more per day, stomach irritation and vomiting may occur.

Recommended Daily Allowance (RDA) and Therapeutic Doses

A common question about RDAs and therapeutic doses for various supplements is: Why is there such a wide discrepancy between the two? The RDAs are the minimal amounts needed to maintain health when consumed by a healthy individual who eats a well-balanced diet. Most medical experts believe these standards are unrealistic because few people meet them and because the RDAs do not consider factors that impact how the body absorbs and uses nutrients. Those factors include illness, use of drugs (legal and illegal, alcohol, and tobacco), emotional stress, pollutants, dietary differences, and physical activity level.

Therapeutic doses are those that support optimal health and/or treat specific conditions. Table 4.1 lists various nutrients, their RDA, and the recommended therapeutic dosage. For nutrients not assigned an RDA, the EDMR, or Estimated Daily Minimum Requirement, is given.

TABLE 4.1 SUPPLEMENT GUIDELINES FOR OPTIMAL HEALTH

Nutrient	*RDA/EMDA*	*Therapeutic Dosage*
Vitamin A (retinol)	4,000–5,000 IU	5,000–10,000 IU
Beta-carotene	2.4–3 mg	5,000–25,000 IU
Vitamin D	400 IU	100–400 IU
Vitamin E (d-alpha tocopherol)	400 IU	400–1,200 IU
Vitamin K	65–80 mcg	60–900 mcg
Vitamin C	60 mg	500–9,000 mg
Vitamin B1 (thiamin)	1.1–1.5 mg	10–100 mg
Vitamin B2	1.3–1.7 mg	10–100 mg
Vitamin B6	1.6–2 mg	25–100 mg
Niacin	15–19 mg	10–100 mg
Biotin	30–100 mcg	100–300 mcg
Pantothenic acid	4–7 mg	25–100 mg
Folic acid	400 mcg	400–1,000 mcg
Vitamin B12	2–2.2 mcg	200–1,000 mcg
Choline		10–500 mg
Inositol		10–500 mg
Boron		1–2 mg
Calcium	800–1,500 mg	250–750 mg
Chromium	50–200 mcg	200–400 mcg
Copper	1.5–3 mg	1–2 mg
Iodine	150 mcg	50–150 mcg
Iron	10 mg	15–30 mg
Magnesium	280–350 mg	250–500 mg
Manganese	2.5–5 mg	10–15 mg
Molybdenum	150–500 mcg	10–25 mcg
Potassium	2,000 mg	200–500 mg
Selenium	55–70 mcg	100 mcg
Silica		200–1,000 mcg
Vanadium		50–100 mcg
Zinc	15–30 mg	15–30 mg

Foods and supplements may be the mainstay of sexual fitness, but the natural world also offers many wonderful opportunities to boost that fitness. In the next chapter you will discover the sexual power of plants and homeopathic remedies.

CHAPTER FIVE

Plant-Plus Power: Herbs and Homeopathy

The natural world offers many ways to attain and maintain sexual fitness. At this very moment, an herb growing in your garden, a "weed" sprouting in your yard, or a flower blooming in the field down the street may hold the promise of more sexual vitality, a remedy for impotence, a tonic to soothe anxiety about sexual performance, or a formula that boosts sexual desire. If you prefer to have your natural remedies "ready made," go to the shelves of your local pharmacy, natural food store, or supermarket: They hold the tea, capsules, tablets, extracts, or powders that can provide the same relief the homemade formulas give you.

This chapter takes you on a journey through the herbal formulas and homeopathic remedies that can improve your sexual fitness. If you are unable to find the remedies locally, Appendix B lists a variety of mail-order locations. It is recommended that you consult with a health practitioner who is knowledgeable about the type of formulas you choose to take. Naturopaths, homeopaths, and herbalists as well as some physicians and pharmacists, especially compounding pharmacists, may be of assistance.

The Power of Herbal Medicine

For thousands of years, cultures around the world have appreciated and benefited from the medicinal and healing powers of plants. But it wasn't until recently that scientists and researchers have begun to uncover the scientific basis for the powers of Nature.

Make no mistake: Plants possess some very potent medicinal abilities, and they should not be used lightly or without first investigating their benefits and drawbacks. Herbs can interact with each other and with other substances. When taken as recommended, however, herbal remedies rarely cause side effects, unlike conventional medications. Please consult your physician before you take herbs if you are currently taking any type of drug or have a medical condition.

Foundations of Herbal Medicine

Of the many types of herbal medicine systems practiced around the globe, the most common are the Ayurvedic, Chinese, European, Native American, and Western. In all of them, the word "herb" refers to any plant or plant part that has medicinal or nutritional value. All of the systems also share several common tenets: that plants possess energy which can be used to treat a person/body as a holistic entity; that each person/body has unique and changing needs; and that the effectiveness of the sum of a plant's parts is greater than that of its individual components. It is believed that each herb was created with compounds designed to work synergistically in the healing process. The power of plants and their ability to work without adverse effects lie in this special relationship.

Forms of Herbal Medicine

Herbs and herbal formulas come in many forms, depending on the herb you want to take and the reason you want to use it. For our purposes, the forms you will most likely use are infusions, tinctures, decoctions, and extracts, all of which are explained in the following pages. Ready-to-use herbs and herbal formulas are available in many pharmacies, herb shops, and natural foods stores, or you can buy raw herbs and make your own remedies. The advantages of commercially prepared herbal remedies are convenience and a longer shelf life—usually several months to a year. If you prepare your own remedies, you can choose or perhaps even grow your own herbs, so you know the formulas are fresh, yet you usually must use them within days.

Explanations of the four forms of herbal formulas and basic instructions on how to prepare standard remedies from raw herbs follow. Please use glass or earthenware pots rather than metal for preparing herbs, as metal can contaminate the formulas.

Infusions are made from the flowers, leaves, or other soft parts of a plant. Often they are referred to as "teas" and are prepared in much the same way. To prepare a standard infusion, pour 2 cups boiling water over 2 to 3 tablespoons dried or fresh herb. Steep for at least 10 minutes or overnight in the refrigerator in a tightly covered container. Strain off the liquid and drink the tea hot, warm, or cool, depending on the condition you are treating. Infusions deteriorate quickly, so you will need to make a fresh batch daily and keep it cool. Because some herbal teas have a foreign taste, you may want to add honey, lemon, or fruit juice.

Decoctions are made from the roots, stems, and bark of plants. To prepare a standard decoction, boil 1 ounce herb in 2 cups water in a covered nonmetallic container for 20 to 30 minutes. Strain off the liquid and cool. Because decoctions deteriorate rapidly, keep the preparation refrigerated for no more than two days.

Extracts are a highly concentrated form of an herb's active ingredients and are made from the soft, juicy parts of the plant. Commercially made extracts are readily available, or you can make your own. To prepare an extract, crush the juicy parts of the plant and press out the liquid. For medicinal purposes, 1 ounce extract equals 1 ounce pure dry herb. Because extracts deteriorate rapidly, you will need to make fresh batches as needed.

Tinctures require six weeks to reach full potency. To

prepare a fresh tincture, place 1 ounce dried herb in a dark glass container along with 5 ounces vodka, gin, brandy, grain alcohol, or vinegar. Seal the container tightly, mark the level of the liquid on the outside of the container, and store it in a dark place (a cabinet or closet is good). Shake the container 10 to 100 times every day for six weeks. When the tincture level goes down, add more of whatever liquid you used in order to maintain the original level. At six weeks, strain out the plant parts and store the bottle in a cool, dark place.

Herbs to Charge Your Sexual Batteries

Agnus Castus Berries

One interesting thing about this Mediterranean shrub is that it can both increase and decrease sex drive. That's because it works by bringing hormones back to a normal range. Thus whether you have a low sex drive or an overactive one, agnus castus berries can restore a balance. This quality makes agnus castus berries (*Vitex agnus-castus*) especially helpful in the treatment of premenstrual syndrome (PMS) and menopausal symptoms, many of which are caused by fluctuating hormone levels. It is also reportedly effective in treating female infertility.

How to Take. The berries are used to make a decoction or tincture. Take 1 cup decoction or 20 to 30 drops tincture daily, preferably before breakfast. To prepare a tea, pour 1 cup boiling water over 1 teaspoon ripe berries and steep, covered, for 15 minutes. Drink up to 3 cups per day. The berries also can be used as a seasoning. Use a coffee grinder to grind the berries into a powder that you can sprinkle on food. Use about 1/4 teaspoon daily of this peppery tasting herb.

Note. If pregnant, avoid taking after the third month of pregnancy because it can cause premature milk production.

Aloe Vera

Aloe vera is a plant that has cushiony leaves which contain a gel valued for its healing powers. It is a popular houseplant in the United States and grows in various deserts around the world. Among its many benefits is its use as an antibiotic and anti-inflammatory, which make it useful in the treatment of pelvic inflammatory disease (PID). It can kill bacteria, inhibit the growth of *Candida,* and reduce inflammation.

How to Take. Take 2 ounces aloe vera juice or 1 to 2 tablespoons gel two to three times a day.

Note. Mix with juice to disguise the bitter taste.

Ashwagandha

Ashwagandha (ash-wah-GAHN-dah) (*Withania somnifera*) is an Ayurvedic herb that is used to treat impotence and sterility in men and low sexual desire in both men and women. It also is useful as a treatment for herpes and as an overall reproductive tonic for men and women.

How to Take. Ashwagandha is available as a powder and tincture, both of which are prepared from the roots, berries, and leaves of the plant. A standard remedy consists of 1 teaspoon powder mixed with 1 cup warm rice, soy, or cow's milk taken twice daily.

Astragalus

Astragalus (*Astragalus membranaceas*) is commonly used in Chinese medicine as an antibacterial agent, tonic, diuretic, and stimulant. For sexual fitness it is effective in the treatment of herpes, as the Chinese consider it to be one of the best herbs for boosting the immune system.

How to Take. Add 20 to 30 drops tincture to water two times a day until the infection heals. The tincture can also be added to soup or stew immediately before serving.

Note. Also a good source of the mineral selenium.

Black Cohosh

This herb has estrogenlike qualities and helps relieve symptoms associated with menopause and PMS. Black cohosh (*Cimicifuga racemosa*) stimulates secretion of estrogen and progesterone and promotes a sense of calm.

How to Take. Because this is a powerful herb, it is best taken under guidance of a knowledgeable medical professional. To prepare a decoction, boil ½ teaspoon powdered root in 1 cup water for 30 minutes. Drink up to 1 cup per day, several tablespoons at a time. It is also available in capsules; take according to package directions.

Note. If you experience any of the following symptoms while taking black cohosh, stop taking the herb immediately and contact your physician: nausea, abdominal pain, headache, low blood pressure, reduced heart rate, joint pain.

Brier

Also known as greenbrier, this native North American plant has been used by Native Americans for centuries to increase sexual effectiveness and for strength. It is still used for these purposes, especially among people living in the Southwest and Mexico.

How to Take. The upper part of the plant is dried and powdered to use as a tea, or the roots can be boiled and made into a decoction. It is best to purchase the prepared tea and use as directed.

Note. If found in the wild, this herb has tasty blue berries.

Caraway

Caraway (*Carum carvi*) is native to Asia, Europe, and North Africa but is now widely cultivated. The seeds have a calming and antispasmodic effect that is effective in women with dysmenorrhea.

How to Take. To prepare tea, pour 1 cup boiling water over 1 teaspoon freshly crushed seeds and allow to steep for 10 to 15 minutes. Drink three times a day. If you choose the tincture, take 1 to 4 ml three times a day.

Catnip

Although catnip (*Nepeta cataria*) can intoxicate your kitty, its effect on people is quite the opposite. Catnip is grown in the United States and Europe and is used to ease the nervous tension and pains associated with dysmenorrhea.

How to Take. To make catnip tea, pour 1 cup boiling water over 2 teaspoons dried herb and allow to steep for 10 to 15 minutes. Drink three times a day. If you prefer the tincture, take 2 to 4 ml in water three times a day.

Note. Do not boil catnip.

Catuaba

This South American herb is derived from a tree that grows in Brazil. Catuaba (*Erythroxylum catuaba*) is very popular among the indigenous peoples of the Amazon region, where its ability to stimulate the central nervous system has led the people to use it as an aphrodisiac.

In the United States and Europe, catuaba is used as a general tonic for male sexual functioning as well as to treat impotency, sexual tension, low sex drive, and sexual weakness.

How to Take. Catuaba tea is available commercially; follow package directions for preparation. If using powdered catuaba, mix 0.5 to 2 grams in a beverage and drink daily.

Cinnamon

Since the Crusades, cinnamon (*Cinnamomum zeylanicum*) has been used to stimulate the sexual appetites of men and women. Cinnamon increases circulation, enhances energy, and is said to be successful in treating impotence.

How to Take. Prepare an infusion by mixing 1 teaspoon cinnamon in 1 cup boiling water. Drink it a few ounces at a time throughout the day. Cinnamon is often an ingredient in sex-enhancing tonics.

Note. Cinnamon is considered to be a safe herb. If you use cinnamon bark oil, avoid getting it on your skin, as it is an irritant.

Couchgrass

Also known as twitchgrass and dog grass, couchgrass (*Agropyron repens*) grows in many parts of the world. Its rhizome is used to make remedies that help in the treatment of prostatitis and an enlarged prostate gland. Couchgrass provides a mild diuretic effect and is completely nonirritating to the kidneys and bladder.

How to Take. Place 2 teaspoons cut rhizome in 1 cup water and bring to a boil. Let simmer for 10 minutes. Drink this remedy three times a day. Of the tincture, take 2 to 4 ml in water three times a day.

Crampbark

Crampbark (*Viburnum opulus*) is an aptly named herb, because it helps relieve cramps associated with PMS. It also has a calming effect and helps strengthen the uterus.

How to Take. To prepare an infusion, add 2 teaspoons herb to 1 cup water and bring to a boil, Cover and simmer for 10 to 15 minutes. Drink hot three times a day. For the tincture, take 1/4 to 1/2 teaspoon every four hours or as needed for menstrual cramps.

Note. The fresh berries are poisonous, but the rest of the plant is safe to use.

Damiana

The leaves of this South American shrub are used as a tonic for the reproductive system of both men and women. Its therapeutic qualities are especially suited for impotence, premature ejaculation, and sterility associated with anxiety, especially in men. Alkaloids found in damiana (*Turnera diffusa*) appear to have a testosteronelike effect, and testosterone can increase libido in both men and women.

How to Take. To prepare the tea, place 2 heaping tablespoons dried damiana in 1 cup boiling water. Steep for 3 minutes. Drink 1 cup per day. If you prefer the tincture, use 1 teaspoon twice a day.

Note. Do not take more than the recommended dose, as it can cause liver problems.

Dong Quai

You will find this herb under many names, including Chinese angelica, women's ginseng, and dang gui. The root of dong quai (*Angelica sinensis*) has long been used to help maintain normal functioning of the sex organs in both men and women, regulate hormone levels, treat menstrual problems, and boost sexual desire. Dong quai contains phytoestrogens, plant estrogenic substances that help regulate and balance a woman's estrogen levels, regardless of whether they are too low or too high.

How to Take. Take any of the following forms three

times a day: 1 to 2 capsules (most capsules contain 520 mg) with meals; 1 teaspoon tincture; or 1/4 teaspoon fluid extract.

Note. Avoid if pregnant, as it can stimulate uterine contractions. The Chinese recommend not taking dong quai while menstruating.

Echinacea

Echinacea (*Echinacea purpurea*) is a daisylike plant that grows throughout the United States. It is a powerful natural antibiotic, which can kill many viruses, fungi, bacteria, and protozoa. Pelvic inflammatory diseases, including vaginal infections and chronic vaginitis, respond well to echinacea.

How to Take. Take any of the following three times a day: 0.5 to 1 teaspoon liquid extract; 100 to 250 mg powdered extract; or 1 to 2 teaspoons tincture in water.

Note. May cause gastrointestinal problems in some individuals.

Garlic

One of the most effective and commonly used medicinal herbs in the world is garlic (*Allium sativum*). It can be used to treat conditions as diverse as atherosclerosis, diarrhea, and vaginitis. It has proven to be very effective in treating infections that affect sexual activity, such as PID.

How to Take. Garlic can be used in several ways to treat sexually associated conditions.

- Eat several crushed garlic cloves daily to resolve sexual debility.
- Fresh garlic, eaten daily, helps reduce the occurrence of viral, fungal, and bacterial infections. Thus it helps ward off diseases that can affect sexual function, such as PID.
- To fight viral and yeast infections in the vagina, peel a clove of garlic, wrap it in a piece of gauze, and tie a string to one end. Insert the gauze into the vagina; change the garlic and gauze daily.

Note. Most people experience no side effects. In some cases eating raw garlic may cause stomach irritation.

Ginseng

Ginseng is a widely popular herb that was originally used in the Far East about 5,000 years ago and is still very popular today. For those seeking help with sexual issues, ginseng (the Chinese or Korean ginseng, *Panax ginseng,* is more potent than the Siberian type, *Eleutherococcus senticosus*) may boost sex drive in men. It also is said to rejuvenate fertility, as it increases testosterone levels, sperm formation, and growth of the testes. Ginseng also improves impotence, premature ejaculation, and menopausal symptoms as well as replenishes vital energy.

How to Take. Look for ginseng products that have a standardized amount of active ingredient. If you buy *Panax ginseng,* look for ingredients called ginsenosides. A typical dosage for a supplement that contains a 7 percent ginsenoside extract is 200 mg one to three times a day. For Siberian ginseng, look for eleutheroside E. standardized at greater than 1 percent and take 100 mg three times a day.

To make a revitalizing tonic, prepare the following: 1 ounce powdered ginseng, 4 dried apricots, 8 blanched almonds, 2 pints red wine. Combine all the ingredients in a container with a lid and allow them to stand for two weeks. Strain and drink 2 ounces daily.

Note. Because there is little quality control of ginseng products in the United States, the amount of active components they contain can vary greatly. Buy only standardized preparations that list the percentage of ginsenosides and follow the package directions for dosing. Too much ginseng can cause insomnia, nervousness, irritability, menstrual changes, hypertension, and anxiety.

Horsetail

The dried stems of the horsetail (*Equisetum arvense*) are used to make remedies to treat an enlarged or irritated prostate gland. It can be combined with the herb hydrangea (not covered in this volume) in the treatment of prostate problems. Horsetail also helps relieve symptoms of menopause.

How to Take. Pour 1 cup boiling water over 2 teaspoons dried herb and allow to steep for 15 to 20 minutes. Drink this remedy three times a day. The tincture also can be taken three times a day at a dose of 2 to 4 ml in water each time.

Note. Drink the tea for only three to four days to avoid toxicity.

Lycium Fruit

The lycium (*Lycium barbarum*) plant is a Chinese shrub, also known as wolfberry, that has bright red berries. It has long been used to treat premature ejaculation and impotence.

How to Take. Lycium may be taken as a tincture (1/2 ounce in a little water daily), or the dried fruit may be eaten (1/2 ounce daily). A soup also can be prepared by combining 1 ounce fruit, 3 chopped carrots, and 1 chopped onion. Add these ingredients to 2 cups vegetable broth and simmer until the vegetables are cooked. Cool, place in a blender, and blend. Reheat and eat regularly to revitalize sexual energy.

Oats

Recently both wild oats (*Avena futua*) and cultivated oats (*Avena sativa*) have gained a reputation for assisting with sexual fitness. Oats nourish and restore the reproductive organs and help revive lagging sexual desire in both men and women. Wild oats are preferred over cultivated, and cultivated are more effective than groats, or oat grains.

How to Take. To make a tea, place 2 teaspoons oat straw in 1 cup boiling water. Steep for 15 minutes. Drink up to 3 8-ounce cups per day. To take the tincture, add 20 drops to water and drink every two hours as needed.

Note. The best form to use is oat straw; groats are not as effective.

Peppermint

For relief of symptoms associated with dysmenorrhea, try peppermint (*Mentha piperita*). The fresh or dried leaves and flowers are used to make tea and tinctures.

How to Take. To prepare tea, steep 1 to 2 heaping teaspoons dried herb in 1 cup boiling water for 10 minutes. Drink up to 3 cups a day.

Note. Avoid peppermint if you have a history of miscarriage.

Potency Wood

According to a November 1994 article in the *American Journal of Natural Medicine*, potency wood, also known as muira puama (*Ptychopetalum olacoides*), is a safe and effective remedy to improve sexual desire and sexual function. Potency wood is said to have similar effects as yohimbe (see "Yohimbe," p. 123), although the side effects are usually milder.

How to Take. Boil 2 to 4 tablespoons shaved bark in 2 cups water for 15 minutes. Drink 1 ounce of this formula one to two hours before having sex.

Note. Some people have an allergic reaction to potency wood. Test yourself by scratching a 1/2-inch-long mark on the skin of your arm with a sterilized pin. Do not draw blood. Dab on potency wood extract. If the scratch becomes irritated within one hour, you are probably allergic to the herb.

Pygeum

Pygeum africanum is an African evergreen tree whose bark is used to treat male infertility, benign prostatic hyperplasia (BPH), impotence, and prostatitis. Among native Africans it is used for various urinary disorders.

Many clinical trials have been done using pygeum, and the results show that this herb is very effective in relieving some symptoms of BPH (frequent urinating at night, incomplete emptying of the bladder, and difficulty in starting urination). Among men who need to improve their fertility, pygeum is helpful in those who have reduced prostatic secretions. Pygeum increases the amount of seminal fluid, protein, and alkaline phosphatase, the latter two of which need to be at a certain level to support fertility. In men whose impotence is associated with BPH or prostatitis, pygeum can improve the ability to achieve an erection.

How to Take. Look for an extract of *Pygeum africanum* standardized to contain 14 percent triterpenes and 0.5 percent n–7 docosanol. Take 100 to 200 mg per day divided into two doses.

Note. Some men experience gastrointestinal problems such as nausea or stomach pains; however, these symptoms are rarely severe enough to discontinue treatment.

Sarsaparilla

Sarsaparilla (*Smilax sarsaparilla*) is a relative of the asparagus and has a long history of use in Central and South America as a treatment for impotence and sexual diseases. Its effectiveness appears to be linked to substances called steroid saponins, which are the building blocks of the male sex hormones progesterone and testosterone.

How to Take. Take any of the following forms three times a day: 1 heaping tablespoon powdered sarsaparilla stirred into boiling water and taken as a tea; 10 to 30 drops tincture; 2 to 3 teaspoons liquid extract; or 250-mg solid extract.

Saw Palmetto

Saw palmetto (*Serenoa serrulata*) is a powerful herbal remedy for several sexual difficulties, including impotence and enlarged prostate. It is also effective against infertility in both men and women and for loss of sexual desire in women. Saw palmetto works by stimulating the sex hormones.

How to Take. To prepare a decoction, add 1/2 teaspoon crushed berries to 1 cup water. Drink 1 to 2 cups daily. Of the tincture, take 20 to 40 drops in water three times a day; of the extract, 5 to 10 drops in water four times daily. When treating benign prostatic hyperplasia, saw palmetto can be taken every hour during the inflammatory stage. Saw palmetto is also available in standardized capsules. Take according to package directions. For best results, Michael Murray, N.D., recommends taking 160 mg fat-soluble saw palmetto extract standardized to consist of 85 to 95 percent fatty acids and sterols.

For prostate problems try this special remedy. You will need fresh nettle roots, either those you dig up yourself or from an herbalist. Nettle is easy to grow in your home or garden. Dig up two or three handfuls of fresh nettle roots and wash them carefully. Chop into fine pieces, place them in a jar, and cover them with saw palmetto tincture. Allow the roots to steep for two weeks, and shake the jar well every few days. After two weeks, strain and bottle the tincture. Use 30 drops three times a day.

Schisandra Berries

The schisandra (*Schisandra chinensis*) is an ornamental vine that grows in China. Its berries are used to restore libido in both women and men.

How to Take. Schisandra is available as a tincture and dried berries. Take 1 teaspoon tincture three times daily, or prepare a decoction from the dried berries and take ½ ounce daily.

Skullcap

The purple-flowering plant skullcap (*Scutellaria lateriflora*) reportedly can help men and women who are infertile and men who suffer with premature ejaculation. It has the ability to ease nervous tension, relieve depression, and calm the nerves.

How to Take. Use 1 teaspoon dried leaves in 1 cup boiling water. Allow to steep for 10 to 15 minutes. Take 2 tablespoons as needed. If you use the tincture, take 20 drops in water or juice up to three times a day.

Valerian

This native of North America and Europe has a long reputation as a sedative. For this reason valerian (*Valeriana officialis*) sometimes is used to treat premature ejaculation. Valerian consists of substances that act on the same areas of the brain as do Valium and other sedatives, yet the herb does not have the side effects of these drugs (morning "hangover" feeling, mental fogginess, and dependency).

How to Take. Standard doses include a single daily dose of any of the following: 1 to 2 grams dried root as a tea; 1 to 1½ teaspoons tincture; ½ to 1 teaspoon fluid extract; or 150 to 300 mg valerian extract (0.8 percent valeric acid).

Note. If you experience morning sleepiness, reduce the dose.

Yohimbe

Yohimbe (*Coryanthe yohimbe*) has gained popularity as a treatment for impotence for men and as a libido enhancer for both men and women. These claims have been verified by many studies, which show that the herb increases blood flow to the penis and clitoris and also causes the veins to constrict.

Yohimbe is obtained from the bark of a West African tree called the yohimbehe. The bark contains several alkaloids that produce the herb's stimulating effects. One of the alkaloids, yohimbine, has been approved by the Food and Drug Administration (FDA) as a treatment for impotence.

Yohimbe can cause mild visual and auditory hallucinations, which often are accompanied by weakness of the limbs, chills, dizziness, anxiety, nervousness, and nausea. This is followed by a relaxed, physical sensation. Although the body is relaxed, the herb also prompts erection of the sex organs. All of these effects can last from two to four hours.

How to Take. Yohimbe can be purchased as an herbal remedy and by prescription in drugs such as Yocon. To prepare an infusion, add 1 ounce dried herb to 2 cups boiling water. Boil for 3 minutes, then simmer for 20 minutes. Strain the tea and sip it about one hour before you want it to take effect.

Yohimbe is also available in capsules and in tincture form. Take 15 to 20 drops tincture in water or a 250- to 500-mg capsule once daily.

Note. Yohimbe comes with many warnings. Because nausea is a frequent side effect, add 1,000 mg liquid vitamin C to the tea or take a vitamin C supplement along with your dose. Vitamin C also helps the body better assimilate the yohimbe.

Yohimbe is an MAO (monamine oxidase) inhibitor, and its use can result in a dramatic drop or increase in blood pressure if it is taken along with tranquilizers, narcotics, antihistamines, sedatives, large amounts of alcohol, or dairy products. No other drugs should be taken within 10 hours of taking yohimbe.

As mentioned, the alkaloids in yohimbe can cause mild hallucinations, often accompanied by chills, dizziness, anxiety, nausea, weak limbs, and nervousness.

Yohimbine manufacturers recommend that the following people should not use the herb because it can cause significant side effects: women; individuals with a history of heart or kidney problems; people with diabetes, hypertension, or hypotension; elderly people; persons with duodenal or gastric ulcer; and people with psychiatric conditions.

HERBAL SOAK FOR VAGINAL INFECTIONS

This herbal formula can be used both as a female douche and as a soaking solution for the penis when the woman has a vaginal infection, such as candidiasis or chlamydia. In these situations, it is important for both partners to treat and cure the infection, as sexual intercourse during this time can keep reinfecting the woman.

The soak/douche consists of equal parts of chaparral, lavender, sage, and yarrow made into an infusion. The mixture should be as warm as is comfortable. Strain the infusion through cotton muslin cloth before use. Men should soak both the penis and the testicles. If using a bowl or wide-mouthed jar is not comfortable, try a sitz bath. The soak and douche should be done two to three times a day for a day or two beyond the time all symptoms stop.

Homeopathic Remedies

Homeopathy (*homeo* [from the Greek] means like; *pathos,* disease) is a holistic treatment approach that is based on the principle that taking a minute amount of a substance that causes adverse effects when given in larger doses can promote healing. The eighteenth-century physician Samuel Hahnemann, who founded homeopathy, believed that the body can heal itself if it is given the appropriate natural remedies to assist it. Remedies are chosen based on an individual's entire being—physical, mental, emotional, and spiritual—and not just on symptoms, so two people with the same physical condition will likely have different remedies.

Homeopathy is a bioenergy medicine, which means it has an effect on the vital force, also known as the life force or chi. The vital force has a natural tendency toward balance and health, and homeopathic remedies help the body return to that state of health and support the body's ability to prevent illness. Because these remedies essentially have no side effects, they can be used safely along with allopathic (conventional) medicines.

Of the more than 2,000 homeopathic remedies, only about 200 are used regularly. Most remedies are derived from plants; others are prepared from minerals or animal products.

How Homeopathic Remedies Work

Researchers are not sure exactly how homeopathy works. Those who practice and use homeopathy explain that the remedies promote healing by restoring and rebalancing an individual's energy. The secret apparently lies in how remedies are made. The process goes something like this. A ground-up portion of the chosen substance is combined with alcohol or water. This mixture steeps for two weeks and is then filtered. The remaining fluid is called the mother tincture. The tincture then is repeatedly shaken vigorously and diluted with alcohol or water until the desired potency is reached. According to homeopathic principles, this process of diluting the remedy, called potentizing, actually makes it more potent rather than less.

One explanation for this claim comes from quantum physics. All physical objects are composed of energy, and as objects move, they leave behind a trail of energy. As a remedy is repeatedly diluted, the molecules of the substance may disappear but the trail remains, at an extremely high energy level. This high energy level accounts for the remedy's high potency.

The healing process in homeopathy, which is called Herring's Law of Cure, occurs from the inside toward the outside; from the most important organs toward the least important, or from the top of the body to the bottom; and in the reverse order in which the symptoms appeared. When a new symptom replaces a primary one, you have reached a new "layer" of healing. Then you can choose a new remedy to balance the new symptom.

How to Take Homeopathic Remedies

In the following list of homeopathic remedies, you will notice numbers such as "6c" and "30c." These numbers indicate the remedy's potency. The strength increases as the number increases; thus 30c is stronger than 6c. The "c" refers to the centesimal ("hundred") scale and indicates how the remedy was diluted. A 1c remedy is 1 part substance and 99 parts water or alcohol. Dosages of 6c and 30c are the most widely prescribed in the United States.

Consider these factors when taking homeopathic remedies:

- The remedies and dosages in the remedies section are suggestions only, meant to guide you in choosing remedies for yourself and your partner. It is always wise to consult a homeopath or other knowledgeable professional.
- If your symptoms worsen after taking a remedy, you may be experiencing "proving." This feeling should disappear soon. Proving occasionally occurs when people take a potency that is too high for them. If proving occurs, consult with your homeopath and take a lower dose.
- You can purchase ready-made homeopathic remedies as tablets, teas, extracts, tinctures, and creams. Many pharmacies and health food stores carry homeopathic remedies, or you can buy them from your homeopath.
- Before you take a homeopathic remedy, avoid putting anything into your mouth for at least 10 minutes, including food, gum, beverages, toothpaste, tobacco smoke, or mouthwash.
- Do not take conventional medications, such as aspirin, cough medicine, or laxatives, while you are using homeopathic remedies. If you are taking a prescription medication, talk with your physician before you start the homeopathic remedy.
- Homeopathic remedies can be taken without

water. Place the tablets or drops on or under your tongue; this allows absorption to occur through the mucous membranes of the mouth.

• During a course of homeopathic treatment, avoid drinking coffee, even decaffeinated. Coffee can impede the benefits of many remedies.

Choosing a Remedy

Select a remedy that best matches your symptoms and personality. Take that remedy until your primary symptom disappears and then choose the most appropriate

---

THE RULE OF THREE: HOW TO TAKE HOMEOPATHIC REMEDIES

A single homeopathic dose can be defined as any of the following:

- 5–10 drops
- 15–20 granules
- 2–3 tablets

For severe symptoms: Take one dose every 30 to 60 minutes for three doses. Repeat as needed for up to 24 hours until symptoms improve to moderate or mild.

For moderate symptoms: Take one dose every 3 hours for one day until symptoms improve to mild.

For mild symptoms: Take one dose every 6 hours. Repeat as needed for up to 10 days.

---

remedy for the next symptom if one occurs. The Rule of Three dosage guidelines shown in the box on p. 129 can help you determine how to take your dose.

HOMEOPATHIC REMEDIES FOR SEXUAL HEALTH

Aconite

Indication: Pelvic inflammatory disease.

Personal Traits: Vivid imagination, apprehensive, impatient, fear of crowds.

Major Symptoms: Headache with nausea after rising; hot, red face; inflamed eyes with swollen lids; earache; red, dry throat; vomiting with sweating and increased urination; scanty, hot urine that is painful to pass; spine feels bruised and stiff; hot, dry skin intolerant of warmth. Symptoms improve when person is in fresh air or has rested; worse at night and in warm places.

Dose: 30c three to four times a day until symptoms improve

Agnus

Indication: Impotence.

Major Symptoms: Strong sexual desire but impotent; erection not firm enough for penetration; general weakness; depression; testicles and penis feel cold to the individual; recent onset of erection difficulties.

Dose: 30c every 12 hours for five days.

Apis

Indications: Pelvic inflammatory disease, painful intercourse.

Personal Traits: Restless, awkward, indifferent, tearful.

Major Symptoms: Swollen genitalia; ovarian pain with painful periods; confused headache with vertigo, which improves with walking; swollen eyelids; swollen, red nose; sore gums; difficulty swallowing; sore, bruised abdomen; sore, sensitive skin with pricking pains. Symptoms improve in open air and with cold baths; worsen in heat, when touched, and in late afternoon.

Dose: 30c four times a day for one week.

Argentum Nitricum

Indications: Prostate disorders.

Personal Traits: Apprehensive, nervous, melancholic, impulsive, intolerant of heat.

Major Symptoms: Erection lost on penetration; lack of sexual desire; pain on intercourse; throbbing headache or dull, aching head relieved by tight binding; tender, bleeding gums; great desire for sweet foods; watery diarrhea; backache relieved by standing or walking. Symptoms improve in fresh air, in the cold, and after belching; worsen at night, with warmth, and after eating, especially cold foods.

Dose: 6c taken four times a day up to 21 days.

Aurum Metallicum

Indication: Painful intercourse.

Personal Traits: Oversensitive to noise and pain, depressed.

Major Symptoms: Depression; severe headaches that are worse at night; eyes sensitive to light; foul breath; rapid irregular pulse. Symptoms better in the summer, in the fresh air, and with cold applications; worse in cold damp weather and from sunset to sunrise.

Dose: 6c three times a day as needed.

Baryta Carb

Indication: Prostate disorders.

Personal Traits: Shy, upset by strangers, poor memory, thin build.

Major Symptoms: Enlarged prostate gland; frequent urge to urinate; slow urine stream; cold accompanied by swollen upper lip and nose; dry cough worse when weather changes; palpitations; flatulence and indigestion; painful abdomen after eating; swollen neck glands; cold clammy feet. Symptoms better when walking in the open air; worse in cold, damp environment.

Dose: 6c four times a day up to 21 days; or 12c twice a day until improvement is seen.

Belladonna

Indications: Dysmenorrhea, painful intercourse.

Personal Traits: Sturdy build, vigorous mind.

Major Symptoms: Cramping pain worse just before periods and worse when walking; tender abdomen during periods with tearing or heavy pains in womb that are worse when lying down; headache before periods; hot, flushed skin; heavy periods with clotting; mental sluggishness; throbbing headache made worse by sun, cold, menstruation, and movement. Symptoms better in darkness and when bending the head back; worse in bright light, when touched, with pressure, and in the cold.

Dose: For dysmenorrhea: 30c every 12 hours for five days; for painful intercourse: 30c four times a day for one week.

Calcarea

Indication: Painful intercourse.

Personal Traits: Thin, dark hair; long legs; people who are uncertain about what they want.

Major Symptoms: Painful womb before and at start of period, accompanied by nausea; sadness, dullness, and indifference; headache before periods; painful breasts before periods with swelling; backache; clammy, sticky skin; tendency to gain weight; nervousness, restlessness. Symptoms better in dry, warm weather; worse in damp, cold weather, when lifting things, and with worrying.

Dose: 30c every hour up to 10 hours.

Causticum

Indications: Loss of libido, dysmenorrhea.

Personal Traits: Dark hair, sallow skin, dark eyes, rigid thinking.

Major Symptoms: Loss of sexual desire; vagina feels raw and sore. For dysmenorrhea: cramping pain before and during periods; cutting, tearing pain in womb during periods; depression; irritability before periods; suspicious and mistrustful; acne on face; diarrhea during periods; backache; sweating during periods; weakness and weariness during periods. Symptoms improve with warmth and dampness; worsen with cold, dry wind, coffee, and sweet food.

Dose: 30c; for women with loss of libido: every 12 hours for five days; for dysmenorrhea: every hour up to 10 hours.

Chamomilla

Indication: Dysmenorrhea.

Personal Traits: Sensitive to pain, may hate to be touched, impatient, irritable, sensitive to chills and wind.

Major Symptoms: Abdominal pain before and during periods, vomiting with pain, irritability before periods; depressed and bad tempered during periods; restless, heavy periods with clots.

Dose: 30c every hour up to 10 hours.

Colocynthis

Indications: Pelvic inflammatory disease, dysmenorrhea.

Personal Traits: Reserved, have strong opinions about right and wrong.

Major Symptoms: Severe menstrual cramps, irritability. Symptoms improve with pressure and warmth; worsen when eating or drinking and in cold, damp weather.

Dose: 30c twice a day until symptoms improve.

Conium

Indications: Impotence, prostate problems.

Personal Traits: Aversion to being near people, anxious, difficulty in understanding

Major Symptoms: Headache when waking in the morning; extreme sensitivity to light; frequent, sometimes involuntary urination; sexual nervousness; increased sexual desire but impotent; muscle weakness. Symptoms improve with motion and pressure; worsen when lying down, with physical or mental exertion, and in the cold.

Dose: 30c every 12 hours for five days.

Graphites

Indications: Premature ejaculation, pelvic inflammatory disease.

Personal Traits: Dark hair, coarse features, do manual labor outside.

Major Symptoms: Sore vagina; yeast infection worse premenstrually; ulcers on labia; irritating discharge; itchy vagina premenstrually; burning pain in vagina; difficulty concentrating; depression; increased appetite; hair loss; numbness and cramps in hands and feet; intolerance to bright light; swollen glands; cold sores; premature or no ejaculation; aversion to intercourse. Symptoms improve after sleep; worsen after eating cold, sweet food.

Dose: 12c three times a day until improvement is seen.

Lycopodium

Indications: Impotence, prostate disorders, premature ejaculation, dysmenorrhea, pelvic inflammatory disease.

Personal Traits: Firm handshake; lean, haughty air; stooping posture; sallow skin; tend to be teachers, politicians, priests, or lawyers.

Major Symptoms: For impotence: enlarged prostate gland; involuntary emission of semen; complete inability to have an erection, which causes depression. For prostate disorders: back pain before urinating that goes away afterward; need to strain to get urination to begin; urine has heavy red sediment; need to urinate often during the night. For premature ejaculation: increased desire for sex along with a lack of self-confidence and the expectation to fail. For dysmenorrhea: pain in womb before periods; nausea during periods, depression, irritability, and weepiness before periods; suspicious and mistrustful; sluggish brain; headache and bloated abdomen before periods; migraine and backache during periods; clammy and sticky, trembling before periods—worse in the cold. For PID: yeast infection—worse during stress; irritating vaginal discharge—worse after periods with itching; weepiness before and after periods; difficulty concentrating; anxiety; dizziness; increased appetite; frequent urination, chronic cystitis; genital warts; backache; neck stiffness; swollen fingers; dry and itchy skin.

Dose: For impotence and premature ejaculation: 30c every 12 hours for five days; for prostate disorders: 12c twice a day until improvement is seen; for dysmenorrhea: 30c every hour up to 10 hours; for PID: 6c six times a day for up to five days.

Mercurius

Indications: Pelvic inflammatory disease (yeast infection).

Personal Traits: Light-haired, slow speech, slow reactions.

Major Symptoms: Very irritating, stringy, offensive discharge with marked itching and burning soreness of vagina; itching in vagina before periods; burning discharge; inflammation of vulva; chronic headache; dull aching pain in abdomen; frequent urination; genital warts; tender breasts; swollen fingers; itchy skin; wariness, chills alternating with sweats; neuralgia; burning pain over left temple; congestive, constricting headache. Symptoms improve with rest and warmth; worsen with temperature changes, dampness, and at night.

Dose: 6c four times daily up to 14 days.

Nux Vomica

Indications: Premature ejaculation, dysmenorrhea.

Personal Traits: Tend to overindulge in alcohol, tobacco, and rich food; overly sensitive to light, noise, and odors; impatient and quick to blame; competitive; easily chilled.

Major Symptoms: For premature ejaculation: anxiety and tension around premature ejaculation; short-tempered; impatient; crave excitement. For dysmenorrhea: cramping pain and tenderness in abdomen, which improves when bending over; nausea and vomiting with pain and irritability before and during periods; acne on face; heavy periods; prolonged periods that arrive early; weakness and exhaustion during periods. Symptoms better in the evening, after rest, and in damp weather; worse in the morning; in cold, dry weather; and after eating.

Dose: For premature ejaculation: 30c every 12 hours up to five days; for dysmenorrhea: 30c every hour up to 10 doses.

Phosphoric Acid

Indications: Low libido in women; premature ejaculation.

Personal Traits: Mild, yielding temperament; strong constitution that has been undermined by depression, illness, or grief.

Major Symptoms: Semen is discharged before or shortly after erection occurs; rash on scrotum; craving for juice and cold milk; dry, cracked lips; frequent, profuse urination, especially at night; apathy and indifference; arms and legs feel weak. Symptoms better in warm environment and with sleep;

worse after sexual exertion and with wind, standing, and sitting.

Dose: For low libido in women: 30c every 12 hours for five days; for men: 12c three times daily until symptoms improve.

Pulsatilla

Indications: Prostate disorders, dysmenorrhea.

Personal Traits: Shy, gentle, fair skin, plump, changeable.

Major Symptoms: For prostate disorders: thick, yellow discharge from penis; urgent need to urinate; headache; dry mouth and lips; backache. For dysmenorrhea: delayed, dark, intermittent periods; chills that increase as pain increases; pain causes patient to double over; vomiting or nausea with pain in womb during periods, which worsens with walking; irritable; dullness and indifference. Symptoms better in open air and after eating cold food and drinks; worse in wet, windy weather, in warm rooms, and after eating hot or rich food or drinks.

Dose: For prostate disorders: 30c three times a day until improvement is seen; for dysmenorrhea: 30c every 2 to 3 hours up to 10 doses as soon as pain begins.

Sepia

Indications: Loss of libido, painful intercourse.

Personal Traits: Tall, lean, narrow hips; soft facial features; dark hair, sallow skin; crave spicy or sour foods and chocolate.

Major Symptoms: For loss of libido: indifference to sex; irritability; feel chilly; feel invigorated after brisk exercise. For painful intercourse: heavy dragging sensation in lower abdomen; during intercourse, pain shoots through vagina and uterus to navel. General symptoms: headache with nausea; extreme sensitivity to odors; pale lips, coated tongue, and sour taste in mouth; irritability; repressed anger, fear, and despair. Symptoms improve with exercise, warmth, and sleep; worsen with cold air, dampness, and in the morning and evening.

Dose: For loss of libido, 30c every 12 hours up to five days; for painful intercourse: 6c every 4 hours up to two weeks.

Staphisagria

Indications: Painful intercourse, especially vaginismus (involuntary closing of the vaginal opening).

Personal Traits: Tend to repress emotions, especially when in love; mild exterior hides emotional turmoil.

Major Symptoms: Sensitive vulva and vagina; pain in ovaries during intercourse. General symptoms: headache made worse by yawning or excessive sexual activity; painful eyeballs; eczema; intense appetite, even when full; cystitis; impatience; easily wounded by words. Symptoms improve with warmth and after sleep; worsen with smoking, anger, grief, and being touched.

Dose: 6c every 4 hours up to two weeks; for vaginismus: 30c every 12 hours for five days.

Now that you've had an opportunity to sit back and sample some of nature's aids for sexual fitness, it's time to get moving. Yes, it's time for exercise, but not just the types of exercise you read about in most books. Get ready for fitness with a twist!

CHAPTER SIX

Are You Fit for Sex?

You've probably never exercised like this before! This chapter explores some familiar—and perhaps some unfamiliar—ways to build sexual prowess and pleasure by exercising with your partner and explains some special exercises you can do alone to strengthen and tone your sexual muscles. Exercise *can* feel good and be *sexy,* and this chapter shows you how. There's also a quick review of the benefits of traditional aerobic exercise.

Aerobic Power = Staying Power

Remember the old adage from elementary school science class that "energy begets energy"? It holds true for sex as well as for physics. Lack of exercise can lead to low energy levels, chronic fatigue, and loss of interest in sex. If you follow a routine aerobic program for only a few months, you will likely notice many of the following benefits.

- Improved cardiovascular fitness and blood flow. A strong heart and good circulation, especially to the genital area, helps promote sexual response.
- Better flexibility. As you become more flexible, you and your partner may want to try new positions.
- Increased sensitivity to how the body functions. When you are more in tune with your body, you can appreciate a greater awareness of pleasure throughout your body.
- Improved muscle tone. Orgasm is the result of muscle contractions that occur in a wavelike motion. Well-toned muscles can result in more intense orgasms.
- Improved self-image and self-esteem. When you look good, you feel good about yourself. Men and women who don't like their body often find it hard to enjoy sex. When you like your body, you project those positive feelings to your partner as well.
- Increased overall strength. Improved strength allows you to ward off fatigue and increase your sexual fitness.
- Improved production of testosterone. This male hormone is associated with increased sexual desire in both men and women.

- Increased production of endorphins, the body's natural painkillers. Endorphins promote a natural "high," often referred to as the "runner's high," which is accompanied by reduced anxiety and stress.
- Possible weight loss. Dropping pounds can not only make you look better and feel better about yourself, it also can give you more sexual stamina and improve overall health.
- Boost in the production of DHEA, a hormone secreted by the adrenal gland. Some experts believe it increases sexual function and overall energy level.
- Increased production of estrogen in women, which helps keep the vaginal tissues moist and supple, prevents heart disease, and increases bone density.

Too Much of a Good Thing

For optimal sexual fitness, don't overdo it! Too much exercise lowers testosterone levels and sex drive in men and women. Women who exercise to excess (competitive runners and gymnasts) may stop menstruating because their hormone system shuts down to protect the body from damage. Moderation is the key. Many doctors and fitness experts recommend 20 to 30 minutes of aerobic activity four to five days a week to maintain health and weight.

Aerobics Should Be Fun

The biggest problem with exercise is that people view it as a chore, a have-to-but-don't-want-to activity. Choose an activity that is fun for you—and your partner, if you can exercise together. Make a date to walk, jog, run, bike, ski, swim, or take an aerobics or Jazzercize class together as often as possible. Find an exercise buddy for times your partner can't join you.

An often-overlooked aerobic exercise that is also a great prelude to sex is dancing. To be aerobic, you need to choose dances and music that get your heart pumping. This can include everything from fast-paced country and western music to calypso and reggae; from belly dancing to square dancing to free-form fast dancing. You and your partner can take dancing classes or simply let loose in the privacy of your home.

The Four Muscle Groups

You can boost and improve your sexual fitness by exercising certain groups of muscles. No, not your biceps or quadriceps, although it can't hurt to build them up as well. But if you want to focus on the muscles that can heighten your sexual pleasure, the four groups you need to work on are the pubococcygeal muscle, the uterine muscle, the diaphragm, and the pelvic muscles.

Pubococcygeal Muscle

In both men and women, the pubococcygeal (PC) muscle runs between the tailbone in the back and the pubic bone in the front. It is the muscle you use to stop the flow of urine. It is the same muscle for which gynecologist Arnold Kegel, M.D., developed exercises in the 1940s to help his patients cope with incontinence. A by-product of his efforts was the discovery that strengthening this muscle also improved sexual pleasure and toned the prostate gland. His simple set of exercises (explained in the box, pp. 145–146) are called Kegel exercises, and they have been helping men and women enhance their sexual fitness ever since.

To help identify your PC muscle, wait until you need to urinate, then sit on the toilet with your knees apart (for women) or stand (for men). Begin to urinate and then try to stop the flow. Allow a bit more urine to flow, then stop the flow again. As you squeeze in the pubic area, you will notice that the region around the anus also tightens. This is the other end of the PC muscle.

If you are a woman, you can use another method to identify your PC muscle. Lie on your back and insert two fingers into your vagina. Pretend you are trying to stop the flow of urine. You should feel the PC muscle constrict around your fingers as well as a tightening around the anus.

Both men and women can benefit from strengthening their PC muscle. Kegel exercises increase blood flow to the genital area, help keep the prostate supple, and strengthen the muscles that support the sex organs. Women who keep these muscles toned can increase the intensity and pleasure they receive from a clitoral orgasm, while men can control their erection to delay ejaculation and increase arousal. According to Alice Ladas, Ed.D., a sex therapist and the coauthor of *The G-Spot,* women who want to experience vaginal orgasms can greatly benefit from strengthening their PC muscle. "Research shows that the weaker your PC muscles, the less likely you are to be vaginally orgasmic," she says. Another coauthor of *The G-Spot,* John D. Perry, Ph.D., believes that many women who say they are not having orgasms are actually having them but cannot feel them because their PC muscle is weak.

Uterine Muscle

Exercising your uterine muscle can enhance the intensity of your orgasms. You can do this exercise in bed, before you go to sleep at night and when you wake up in the morning. While lying on your back, bend your knees and keep your feet flat on the bed. Let your knees fall comfortably to either side. Press the small of your back into the bed and tighten the muscles in your lower abdomen. If you feel air entering and leaving your vagina, you have found the uterine muscle. Keep contracting the muscles and moving the air in and out for a count of 10 to 15. Do this exercise twice a day. Don't do this exercise if you are pregnant.

KEGEL EXERCISES

Kegel exercises can be done just about anywhere and anytime: while you sit in traffic, watch television, work at your desk, or wait in line at the grocery store. For best results, exercise your PC muscle regularly. To get into the habit of doing Kegels at least twice a day, you may want to exercise before you get out of bed in the morning and when you go to bed at night, or on your commute into and from work. Some experts recommend doing them four to five times a day to experience peak sexual fitness.

Kegel exercises are done in three parts. Don't worry if you can't hold a clench for as long as mentioned in the instructions. Like any other muscle, the PC can get tired and will do so quickly in the beginning, especially if you're not used to working it so hard. Do each of the three parts during each exercise session.

1. Slow Clench: Squeeze and clench the PC muscle as if you were stopping urine. Hold the clench for a slow count of three, then relax. Repeat nine times for a total of 10 slow clenches.
2. Rapid Clench: Repeatedly clench and relax the PC as rapidly as you can for a count of 10 clenches.
3. Push Out: Bear down with moderate pressure as if you were forcing a bowel movement. This works the tailbone end of the PC as well as a few abdominal muscles. Do this 10 times.

Each of these three exercises makes up one set. You might begin by doing one of each set, four to five times a day, for the first week. Then in week 2, increase the number in each set to 15. In week 3, increase the number to 20, and so on until you reach 30. By that time you should notice a significant improvement in your sexual fitness and satisfaction, and so will your partner! Once your PC muscle is well toned, you can maintain its strength by doing 30 repetitions in each of the three sets about three times a week.

Diaphragm Strength

During sexual intercourse, tightening the diaphragm can increase vaginal sensation because the vagina is pushed toward the penis. You can exercise your diaphragm muscle—the band of muscle located at the lower part of the rib cage—without even leaving your desk.

Sit straight in your chair with your feet flat on the floor and your arms either on the chair arms or at your sides. Lift both feet off the floor, keeping your knees together, about 6 to 8 inches from the floor. Hold for 5 to 10 seconds and breathe normally. Lower your feet to the floor. Repeat this exercise 10 to 15 times twice a day.

Pelvic Muscles

Strong, flexible abdomen, lower back, and buttock muscles are essential if you want control of your pelvic region, which can improve your sexual fitness and satisfaction. The following exercises will increase your range of motion and help you better position your pelvis during sexual intercourse. They take only a few minutes to do. Ask your partner to join you!

Pelvic Rock: Lie on your back with your knees bent and your feet flat on the floor. Slowly rock your pelvis up without lifting the small of your back from the floor. This movement causes your buttock muscles to tighten and your lower back to stretch. Hold the lift for several seconds, then relax. Repeat 10 times.

Tummy Crunch: Lie on your back with your knees bent and your feet flat on the floor. Place your fingers lightly behind your ears and relax your arms. Tighten and pull in your abdominal muscles, then slowly curl your head and shoulders up toward your knees until your lower back is pressed flat against the floor. Hold that position for three to five seconds, then slowly return your upper back and head to the floor, while continuing to contract your abdominal muscles. Repeat 10 times.

Bedroom Workouts for Two

Working out with your sexual partner may be the ultimate way to exercise, and here's why. First, a common complaint about exercise is that it's not fun, but exercising with your partner *is*. Second, many people say they don't feel motivated. You'll have several motivations when you exercise with your sexual partner: Better flexibility and strength means better sexual performance; you'll look and feel better about yourself;

and you can be enticing while you move together. Third, exercising together allows both of you to be intimate with each other without being sexual, unless of course it leads to that!

The bedroom workouts in this section include a series of five stretches, which were chosen because they are easy, effective, and can be done by most people. Stretching from head to toe is an excellent way to release stress and tension, send more oxygen surging through the body, and make the body more supple—all of which improve your sexual fitness. In particular, a strong yet flexible lower back allows you to make the pelvic thrusts and other midbody movements during sexual intercourse that are an important part of sexual pleasure.

The key to doing partner exercises effectively is communication and trust. Because you will be holding on to each other during each exercise, you need to let each other know how far to stretch and when to stop. Do not bounce or pull; ease into each stretch to avoid injury. To improve flexibility for both you and your partner, practice the following sexy stretches as a prelude to lovemaking.

Two-V Stretch (See Figure 6.1)

This stretch works best for partners who are of similar height but is also effective for those who may have a foot or more difference between them. Do this stretch slowly and gently at first until both of you have gained some flexibility.

- Sit on the floor facing each other with your legs extended out in a comfortable V-shape.
- Allow the bottom of your feet to match up with the bottom of your partner's feet. The V-stretch needs to be comfortable for the person with the shorter legs.
- Reach out straight in front of you and grasp each other's hands. While holding hands, slowly and gently lean forward, hold for a few seconds, and then lean back. You may not move more than an inch or two, but you will feel the stretch in the back of your legs.
- Now lean to the right, hold for a few seconds, then lean to the left.
- Try to make a circle: lean forward, to the right, then back, then to the left.
- Repeat the circle several times.

Seated Stretch (See Figure 6.2)

- Sit back to back on the floor with your knees bent and relaxed and your feet flat on the floor. Interlock your elbows with your partner's elbows.
- Slowly lean forward, bringing your head toward your knees. Your partner should relax

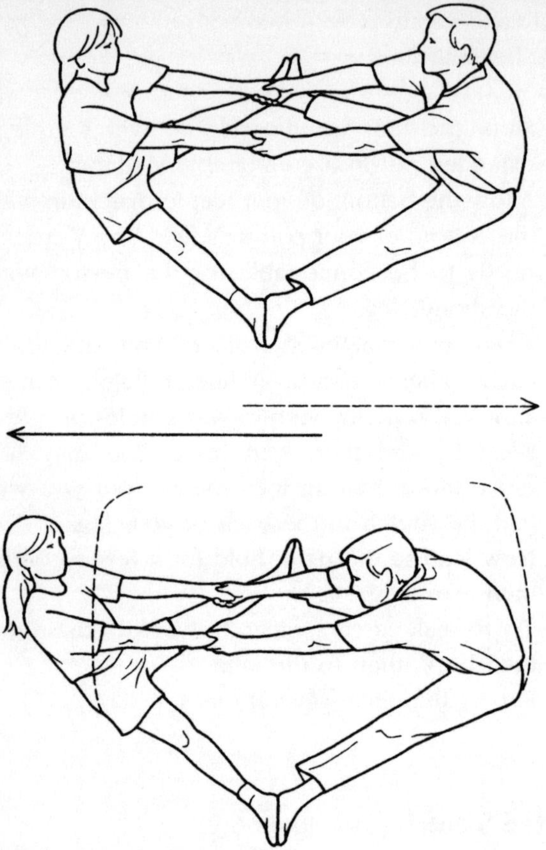

FIGURE 6.1

and allow him- or herself to stretch backward as far as is comfortable.

- Hold the stretched position for five to six seconds.

- Slowly return to the upright seated position. Your partner now repeats the movements.
- Repeat the exercise five to six times. This exercise stretches the lower back and abdominal muscles.

Rock-a-Back (See Figure 6.3)

- Sit on the floor facing your partner. Each of you should have your legs crossed and your knees nearly touching.
- Reach out and grasp each other's forearms where it is comfortable and where it allows both of you to sit up straight and not lean forward.
- Lean back slowly, gently bringing your partner toward you. Keep your buttocks on the floor.
- Hold the stretch for several seconds, then return to an upright sitting position.
- Your partner now repeats the stretch.
- Repeat the exercise five to six times. This stretch limbers up the hips, lower back, and shoulders.

Hip-Knee Stretch (See Figure 6.4)

- Lie down on your back with one leg bent and your foot flat on the floor. Your partner should kneel on the floor at your side.

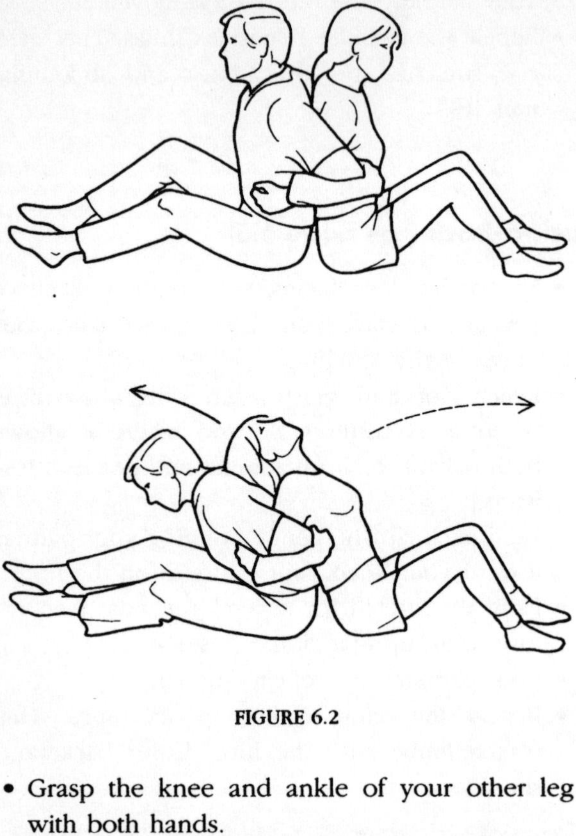

FIGURE 6.2

- Grasp the knee and ankle of your other leg with both hands.
- Your partner should hold the knee and ankle of your bent leg and gently stretch your knee toward your chest while keeping your ankle straight in relation to your knee. Hold this position for 15 seconds.

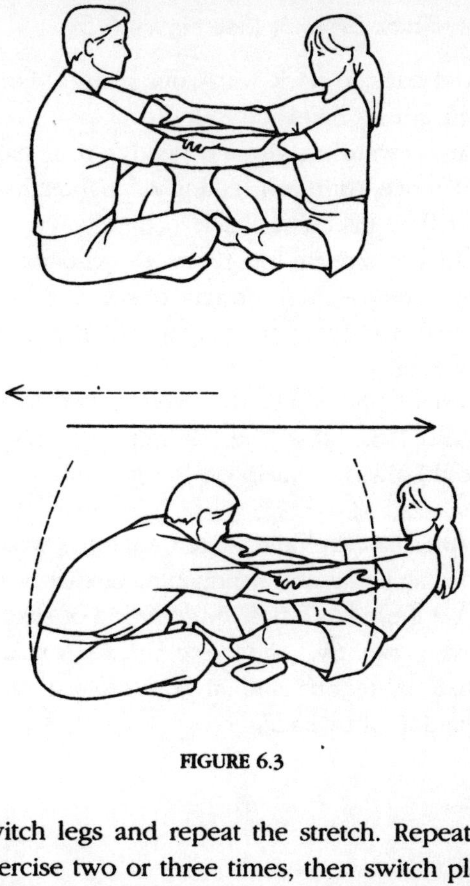

FIGURE 6.3

- Switch legs and repeat the stretch. Repeat the exercise two or three times, then switch places with your partner. This exercise stretches the muscles of the hip.

Back-to-Back Stretch (See Figure 6.5)

- Stand back to back with your partner, holding each other's hands at your sides.
- Lean forward slowly and gently. Your partner will move with you, taking deep breaths and stretching his or her back against yours.
- Hold the stretch for 10 to 15 seconds, then slowly return to an upright position.
- Repeat, with your partner stretching your back this time.
- Alternate and repeat the exercise two to three times. Note that the shorter person's feet should always remain on the ground.

This chapter has explored more traditional Western exercises for attaining and maintaining sexual health and fitness. Yet there is a whole other world of sexual techniques you can try. The next chapter explains the somewhat mysterious and always sensual worlds of Tantric and Taoist sexuality.

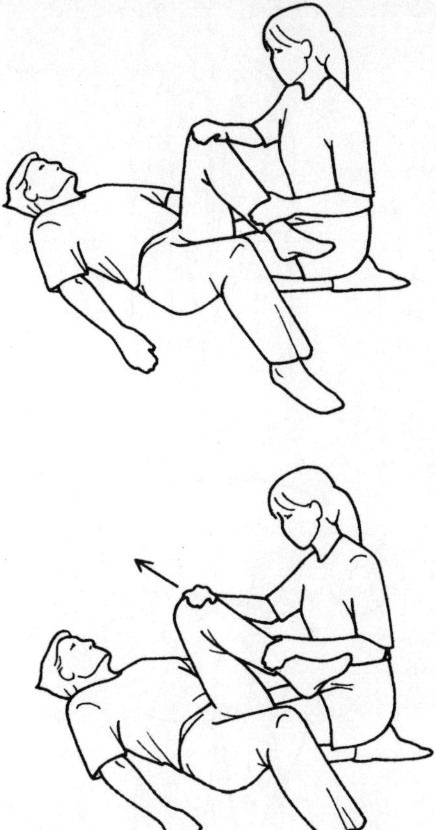

FIGURE 6.4

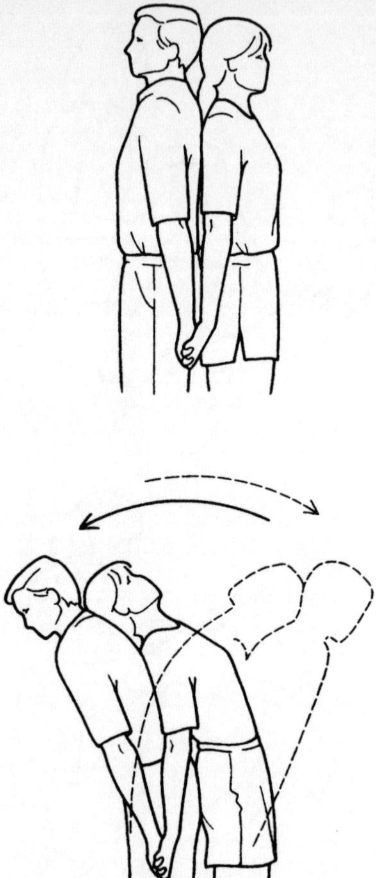

FIGURE 6.5

CHAPTER SEVEN

Eastern Sexual Traditions

Enter the mystical and sexually charged worlds of Tantric and Taoist sexuality. "Tantra" is a Sanskrit word that is associated with an Indian philosophy that is more than 4,000 years old. The word means "the weaving of energy," and the philosophy teaches that people can weave the realities of their entire being into a more interrelated or synergistic whole. On a sexual level, this philosophy is a way of being in love with your partner with your whole heart, mind, and spirit in an atmosphere of openness and trust.

Taoism is Chinese wisdom that also is thousands of years old. Its basic philosophy is that energy and momentum are the sources of all life and that unless humans harmonize with all of the infinite natural sources, they cannot continue to exist. Thus the Taoist way of life teaches people to be natural and completely relaxed, and this philosophy forms the basis of their attitude about sexuality.

Taoist sex exercises are based on ancient erotic rituals and can help people discover the magic of sexual energy. Certain types of Tantric yoga exercises from ancient India and nearly all the Taoist exercises from ancient China were developed solely to help people enjoy longer-lasting, sexually fulfilling lovemaking.

These ways of looking at love and sex are very different from how Westerners, and Americans in particular, are used to thinking about them. According to Dr. John Mumford, author of *A Chakra & Kundalini Workbook,* "the attitude in tantra toward sexual expression is one of liberation and reality rather than repression or suppression," which is how most Americans view sex. Tantric love and the Taoist approach to lovemaking both allow people to harmonize with each other, experience full-body orgasm, and immerse themselves in love and passion.

A Healing Love

Both Tantra and Taoism can be described as prolonged meditation, in which two people connect physically, emotionally, and spiritually and heal each other on all these levels. The healing occurs as couples move away from the expectations associated with the Western approach to sex: "Did you come?" "Did I do it right?" "I don't know how to please my husband." "My penis is too small." "I come too soon." "I can't reach orgasm with my partner." Couples put aside thoughts of goals, quiet the mind, and focus on breathing. They become emotionally and spiritually connected with their partner. This process heals, because it eliminates being set up for rejection, shame, fear, regret, inadequacy, and other negative feelings that go along with performance anxiety and goal setting in sex.

Eastern Sexuality for You

The Tantric and Taoist disciplines both consist of many beautiful yet sometimes complex principles and exercises partners can share. They also include many rituals—a series of symbolic words, songs, movements, gestures, and invocations—that are used to support and advance sexual experiences. Because space does not permit an explanation of these rituals, the techniques presented here have been "westernized" to make them easy to understand and to do. It is hoped that they will not only improve your sexual fitness but also pique your interest to explore them further. (See Suggested Readings for books on Tantric and Taoist sexuality.)

These Eastern approaches to sex seem foreign to Western couples, but many people who try them find they allow them to reach new depths of love, understanding, and connectedness with their partner. The Eastern concept of sexual fitness truly transcends the physical, as the following exercises will demonstrate. Try them with an open mind.

Eastern Sex Exercises

The sex exercises explained next come primarily from the Taoist tradition. Tantric yoga exercises for sexual fitness are discussed in Chapter 8.

Taoist exercises are especially effective at nurturing sexual vitality and allowing individuals to control their sexual fitness and pleasure. This ability to manipulate sexual energy derives from the belief that all of the body's energy (chi, or vital force) travels along invisible pathways called meridians, which cross through the pelvic region. When there is interference (disease, tension, weakness) in that area, the vital force and sexual force weaken or are lost. Taoist exercises strengthen, tone, and revitalize sexual energy in the pelvic region, which in turn improves sexual fitness and helps treat impotence, loss of libido, infertility, prostate disorders, pelvic inflammatory disease, and menstrual problems.

Once the sex glands and organs are recharged by the Taoist exercises, they are able to send that sexual energy throughout the body, healing as it goes, and then storing it in the navel area, or solar plexus. This healing circuit is accomplished by doing Taoist techniques, which involve breathing exercises, imagery, and contracting certain muscles, like the pubococcygeal muscle and the vaginal muscles.

Of the many rituals that are part of Tantric sexual

practices, one of the most basic is the Melting Hug. Couples are encouraged to begin all of their sexual encounters with the Melting Hug as a way to prepare themselves for the loving, mystical experience they are about to share.

MELTING HUG

- You and your partner stand and face each other. Move toward each other slowly as you open your arms and embrace in a tender hug.
- Wrap your arms around each other and make sure your bodies are touching, without undue pressure, at the chest, belly, pelvis, and thighs.
- Continue to hold each other as you focus on your breathing. Feel the warmth of your partner as you each breathe easily and in harmony. Experience the rise and fall of your bodies together as you breathe.
- Hold the Melting Hug for as long as you wish, then separate gently.
- Step back from each other and look into each other's eyes. Silently acknowledge the love, respect, and gratitude you have for each other.

The Melting Hug is also a good way to both begin and end a lovemaking session.

Better Breath, Better Sex

Breath carries the essence of the life force and is necessary for good overall health and sexuality. Yet most Westerners use less than one third of their lung capacity, thereby robbing their sex organs and glands of invigorating and life-sustaining energy. Eastern disciplines practice deep breathing, which sends energy to the pelvic area, the center of sexuality, and energizes the entire body.

Once you learn how to control your breath, you will have control of your sexual energy. Breath control is easy to learn and can be practiced anywhere and anytime, so you can improve your sexual fitness even while sitting at your desk at work or waiting at a traffic light. The Basic Breath, which is explained next, is used in yoga, with Tantric and Taoist exercises like those discussed in this chapter, to meditate and simply to relax and ease everyday tension.

BASIC BREATH

- Lie on your back with your knees bent and your feet flat on the floor about hip-width apart. Press the small of your back into the floor. A small pillow or rolled-up towel under your knees can help your back and abdomen relax.
- To gauge your breath, place one hand over your lower abdomen and inhale through your nostrils. Make the breath slow, deep, and even.

Notice how your hand rises. As you exhale your hand should lower.

- With each succeeding breath, try to send more air into your abdomen. Keep your breaths relaxed and deep; do not hold your breath.
- Close your eyes and imagine that each breath is filling your torso, down to your anus. Visualize life-giving air circulating throughout your chest cavity, down to your navel, and then to your pelvis. With each in breath, re-create this picture in your mind. Feel how your genital area expands with sexual energy. Continue to breathe deeply and slowly.
- Once your genital area has been revitalized, send your next breaths down your legs and arms to your toes and fingers. This may prove to be more difficult at first, but with practice you will be able to send breath to those areas as well.
- End your session with a few slow, deep breaths.

Fire Belly Breathing

This breathing exercise lights the fire of desire and raises the sexual energy level of those who practice it regularly. It works by stimulating the sexual energy zone in the pelvic area—from about one inch above the pubic bone to about one and one-half inches below the navel. Because Fire Belly Breathing is a combination of Basic Breath with the motions explained next, do Fire Belly Breathing (below) after you are comfortable doing Basic Breath.

- Stand with feet comfortably apart and knees slightly bent; or sit on the edge of a chair with your back straight. Men should allow their genitals to hang free.
- Rub your palms together until they are hot.
- With your left hand, use a clockwise circular motion to gently rub your lower abdomen. Cover the area from just below the navel to just above the pubic bone. Make 10 or more circles, counting as you go.
- Warm your palms again. Use your right hand to massage the same area, this time using a counterclockwise motion. Make the same number of circles as you did with the left hand.
- Repeat the sequence for each hand as many times as you wish, making sure you do an equal amount in each direction.

Overcoming Impotence: Soft Entry

In the Tao of Loving, or the Taoist approach to sexuality, there is no word for "impotence." What most American men view as a terribly embarrassing problem that causes feelings of helplessness and despair, Taoists see as a natural occurrence and an opportunity to focus elsewhere. They say forget about the erection and concentrate instead on the beauty and magic of your partner's body. After all, they point out that there are many ways to give and receive sexual pleasure. Taoists also accept the fact that it is natural for men not to get an erection always. If a man is experiencing impotency, they suggest the following strategy.

- Explore your partner's body with your hands, tongue, lips, and nose. Give her a slow massage. Smell the heat of her skin. Suck on her toes, her clitoris, and her nipples. Ask her what she wants you to do to arouse her even more.
- As her excitement builds, you may get an erection. If you do, problem solved! If you don't, then try the soft-entry method. The best position for soft entry is either side to side facing one another or with the man on top.
- Continue to caress and stimulate each other. This mutual pleasure-giving time should be done without expectations or time limits. Do not think about what may be, but what is happening at the moment.
- Do not attempt to enter the vagina until it is well lubricated. If there is not enough natural lubrication, use K-Y jelly. Apply the jelly either directly to the vagina or to the tip of the penis.
- Soft entry requires finger dexterity on your part. Relax; it may take a few minutes the first few times you try it. Once you have your penis in your partner's vagina, make a ring with your

fingers at the base of the penis. This forces the upper portion of the penis to become semirigid so you can begin to thrust.
- Keep your finger ring at the base of the penis to allow you to control your thrusts until your penis becomes hard.

The soft-entry technique works for most men who are in reasonably good condition. If you are physically, mentally, or emotionally exhausted, or if your diet and lifestyle are poor, it probably will not work.

Exercise for Desire

To increase sexual desire (with the added benefit of relieving lower back pain), try the Taoist technique called the Kidney Stimulator. This exercise strengthens the kidneys, the adrenal glands, and the entire glandular system. Some Taoist healers also use the Kidney Stimulator to treat premature ejaculation and impotence.

KIDNEY STIMULATOR

- Choose a comfortable place to sit or lie down.
- Rub your palms together until they are hot.
- Place your palms on the small of your back and tilt your upper body forward. Imagine the heated energy from your hands is radiating into your kidneys and adrenal glands.
- Use your palms to massage the small of your

back, both up and down and then in a circular motion.

- Make a loose fist and gently pound the small of your back for about 10 seconds.
- Alternate between massaging and pounding the small of your back for three complete cycles.

Loose and Sexy

A simple but very effective Taoist exercise is the Hip and Sacrum Loosener. Sexual satisfaction and fitness depend on good flexibility and mobility in the hips and sacrum, or tailbone. Many people tend to be stiff in the pelvic region, which limits their ability to become sexually aroused. With regular practice, this exercise can give your hips more swivel and thrusting power. Do it with your partner, so he or she can help stabilize your hips.

HIP AND SACRUM LOOSENER

- Stand with your feet about hip-width apart and knees slightly bent.
- Place your hands on your hips. If your partner is with you, have him or her place his or her hands over yours.
- Focus on moving your sacrum bone forward and back. You can accomplish this by thrusting your pelvis forward and back and allowing your sacrum to follow. Make sure your hips do not move. It may help to place one hand on

your hip and the other on your sacrum to isolate the movement, or your partner can do the same for you. Practice this movement for two to three minutes several times a day.

Sexual Energy Boosters

The Taoists have an exercise known as the Deer, which enhances energy levels and balances the function of the sex glands. When the sex glands operate at their best, you can be at your sexual best as well, with high sexual desire and great vitality. The exercise, which has a version for men and for women, focuses on toning the anal muscles and, in women, the vaginal muscles. Both the Male Deer and Female Deer are typically done in the nude.

The Male Deer. When a man exercises the anal sphincter, the prostate gland, which is located behind the anal muscles, also benefits. Toning of the prostate gland helps prevent prostate disorders such as inflammation and benign prostatic hypertrophy, premature ejaculation, and impotence. Some men claim the Deer can even increase the size of the head of the penis, although this has not been proven.

- Sit on the edge of a sturdy chair and allow your testicles to hang free.
- Rub your palms together until they are very warm.
- Cup your testicles gently with your right hand.

Close your eyes and visualize the heat and energy radiating from your hand to your testicles.

- While keeping your right hand on your scrotum, place your left palm about one inch below your navel. This is your solar plexus, or third chakra. (See the box on chakras, p. 172.) Gently massage the area using a clockwise circular motion. Repeat the massage using a counterclockwise motion. Do the same number of motions in each direction.
- When your palms become cool, repeat the entire sequence, from rubbing your palms together to massaging in both directions in your pubic area, as many times as you wish.
- As you do the massage, squeeze your PC muscles and anal muscles together. Hold the squeeze as long as you can without straining, then relax.
- Repeat the muscle contractions as many times as you can do so comfortably. Always relax after each contraction. The combination of massage and muscle squeezes may feel awkward at first, but with practice you will find it to be easy.
- Practice this exercise twice a day, in the morning and at night.

You may get an erection while doing this exercise. Because the purpose of the Deer is to revitalize the sex organs, having an orgasm would take that energy away. To prevent orgasm, press the thumb of your right hand at the base of your penis. As you apply pressure, massage the pubic bone with your left hand. This will stop the blood from flowing into your penis.

The Female Deer. In women, this exercise tones the reproductive organs and can help prevent organ- and gland-related disorders.

- Sit on a flat surface—the floor, a bed, or a sofa—and place the heel of one foot against your clitoris. If your heel cannot reach, place a hard round ball between your heel and your groin until there is gentle pressure against your clitoris. Maintain that pressure throughout the exercise.
- Rub your palms together until they are very warm.
- Place your hands on your breasts and visualize the heat leaving your hands and radiating into your breasts.
- Rub your palms over your breasts in a circular motion: the right moving counterclockwise and the left, clockwise. Be firm but gentle and continue for a minimum of 36 circles up to no more than 306. This cleansing massage can dissolve lumps.
- Rub your palms together again and place them on your breasts again. This time rub your breasts in the opposite direction. This massage

helps improve firmness and increase breast size.

- While massaging your breasts, tighten your anal and vaginal muscles. Hold the squeeze as long as comfortable. Relax and repeat several times. If at first you cannot massage your breasts and contract the muscles at the same time, simply hold your breasts while squeezing the muscles until you gain more control of your anal and vaginal muscles.

The combination of breast stimulation and pressure against the clitoris stimulates hormone production. Eventually you may want to learn how to send your sexual energy to the rest of your body and enjoy complete body revitalization.

Good control of the pubococcygeal and anal muscles is key in the Taoist sexual discipline, because these muscles allow you to hold on to the sexual energy in your pelvic region. The Taoists believe this is necessary to maintain the vitality of the sex organs, sex hormones, and the body's overall health. However, once you have control of these sex muscles and your sexual energy, you may want to learn how to send that energy to the rest of your body and enjoy complete body revitalization. (See Suggested Readings for books on Taoist sexuality.)

CHAKRAS

The word "chakra" is a Sanskrit term for "wheel." According to Eastern philosophies, each of the seven chakras is an energy center that absorbs and releases the vital life force, or chi. Each chakra has a corresponding endocrine gland and controls a specific region of the body.

Chakra	*Chakra*	*Associated Gland/ Organ*
Crown	7	Pineal
Brow	6	Pituitary
Throat	5	Thyroid/parathyroid
Heart	4	Heart and thymus
Navel/solar plexus	3	Pancreas and adrenal
Spleen	2	Spleen
Root/sacral	1	Sacrum, gonads, ovaries

Healing Pleasures for Women

Self-pleasuring (a more pleasant-sounding term for "masturbation") is a routine part of Tantric and Taoist sexuality. Self-pleasuring is used in various rituals to help individuals and couples improve their sexual relationship. Part of sexual fitness is being free of disease and infections, especially those that affect the sex organs and sexual functioning. An exercise called Sexual Self-Empowerment with a Symbol includes a stage in which women can heal physically, emotionally, and spiritually from pelvic inflammatory disease. It includes the concept of chakras, which is explained in the box on page 172.

SEXUAL SELF-EMPOWERMENT WITH A SYMBOL

- Designate an object to represent the healing force for your vagina. Choose something beautiful, such as a flower, the sunset, or a tropical bird.
- Choose a quiet, comfortable location where you can pleasure yourself without interruption. Set the stage: candles, incense, dim lights, music. Create a healing environment.
- Begin to caress yourself: your breasts, stomach, thighs, and clitoris. Honor your body.
- As you touch your clitoris and vaginal opening, close your eyes (if they are not closed already) and imagine your healing force has entered your vagina and has entered your first chakra. See that flower or sunset as a beautiful healing force that is spreading healing power.
- Continue to pleasure yourself as you imagine the healing image is moving up to your next chakra, carrying light and healing and the center of your sexuality with it.
- Allow your healing force to continue up through each chakra, growing in warmth and vitality, as you continue to honor your body. Feel your sexuality grow more and more beautiful and healthy as it moves up through your chakras.

- When you reach orgasm, send your healing symbol to your seventh chakra and allow its power to radiate throughout your body.

Egg-citing Exercise for Women

A Tantric sexual practice known only to Chinese royalty and courtesans has existed for centuries. It involves the use of a wooden or stone egg, about one inch in diameter, which is inserted into the vagina. Manipulation of the egg by the vaginal muscles builds sexual muscle tone, balances hormone levels, and increases the intensity of orgasm.

Although this practice sounds unusual, it has passed the test of time. Throughout the exercise, keep your vaginal opening contracted or the egg will fall out. This may happen several times until you get more practice. Because many of the muscles you use in this exercise are involuntary, you will be using your mind to control the muscles as much as possible. If the egg gets stuck, it comes out easily if you lie down and squeeze it out.

Here's how you can enjoy this millennia-old tradition, the egg exercise.

- Use a stone or wooden egg one inch or smaller in diameter. Stone eggs are easier to keep clean. Because it is harder to manipulate a smaller egg, you should probably start with the one-inch egg.

- Before inserting a stone egg, boil it for 1 to 2 minutes and let it cool. A wooden egg can be cleaned with a nonirritating, hypoallergenic soap and rinsed thoroughly.
- Your vagina should be lubricated before you insert the egg. You can either stimulate yourself or use a water-based lubricant.
- Insert the egg, wider end first. You may want to stand with one leg up on a chair so you can slide it in easily. Then get into the position to do the exercise: Stand with feet hip-width apart, knees slightly bent, back straight. Stand on a cushioned surface or with a pillow under you in case the egg falls out of your vagina.
- Lift your arms straight out in front of you with palms up and fists clenched.
- Take a deep breath as you contract the muscles that open and close the vaginal opening. Focus on isolating those muscles.
- On your next inhale, concentrate on the muscles higher in the vagina. On the next inhale, tighten the muscles at the top of your vagina.
- Inhale again, and this time squeeze the egg so it moves up into your vagina. Focus on moving the egg up and down your vagina with each inhale. With practice, you should be able to build up speed and rhythm. You also will experience a buildup of sexual energy as you move the egg.

- Once you have learned to move the egg up and down, try moving it left and right. When you master that movement, try combining up and down with left and right.

Practice the egg exercise for two or three minutes several times a week. Over time you will be able to increase the amount of time you can move the egg inside your vagina. Some women advance to two eggs at one time and move them in opposite directions.

Fitness for Your Sex Organs

The following two Taoist exercises were designed to stimulate the sex organs and sex glands in order to increase sexual arousal and pleasure. They are designed for both men and women. If you like, you and your partner can do these exercises together.

Taoist Sex Organ Energizer. Practice this exercise before moving on to the Taoist Energy Transformation technique. In this exercise you will learn how to move your vital energy from your upper body down into your pelvic region.

- Sit in a comfortable straight-back chair or cross-legged on a firm surface with your back straight.
- Inhale deeply through your nose and feel the energy as it enters your throat. Touch the tip of your tongue to the roof of your mouth.

- Imagine the air-energy is a ball. As you swallow the air, send it down to the region between your heart and navel (the third chakra, or solar plexus), then down to your sacrum (first chakra), where you will gather the energy. To help you move the energy, contract your stomach muscles and imagine you are pushing the ball of energy down into your pelvic region.
- To prevent this energy from leaving, squeeze your pubococcygeal and anal sphincter muscles. You may feel your sex organs become full and warm.
- As you exhale, relax and swallow any saliva that has gathered in your mouth.
- Practice lengthening the amount of time you hold the compressions until you can hold them 30 seconds or longer. This exercise revitalizes the entire body and the sex organs in particular. It is regarded as a "battery charger" for sexual fitness.

Taoist Energy Transformation. This technique combines three powerful elements: breath, the PC and anal muscles, and the mind. Its purpose is to build up the concentrated vital energy in the first chakra and then send it throughout the body, where it heals and energizes the entire body and readies it for lovemaking. Be patient with this exercise, as it may take several weeks to master. Follow all the steps in order and enjoy the learning process, as it is a wonderful sexual adventure in itself. Do the exercise in the nude, along with your partner if you like.

- Sit cross-legged on a firm, comfortable surface and rub the palms of your hands together until they are very warm.
- Practice the appropriate Deer exercise. (See pp. 168–171.)
- Caress your body and focus on how the energy and heat from your palms radiate into your body.
- Continue to stimulate yourself until you nearly reach the point of orgasm.
- Just before or in the midst of orgasm, take a deep breath through your nose and tighten all of your muscles, including your pubococcygeal and anal muscles, and your fists, jaw, stomach, and back. Press your tongue firmly against the roof of your mouth.
- Relax all of your muscles except your PC and anal muscles, then clench them all again.
- When you are out of breath, exhale and experience the energy in your sex organs.
- Take another deep breath and hold it. At the same time, squeeze and relax your pubococcygeal and anal muscles in a wavelike motion.

Continue this pumping action, exhaling and relaxing before inhaling and contracting the muscles again.

- As you continue this pumping action, imagine your sexual energy is a shimmering light radiating from your pelvic region.
- After several cycles of squeezing and relaxing, inhale and contract the entire genital and anal region. Send the light down to the area between the anus and the urinary opening. Exhale, and then on your next inhale, pull the light up to the base of your spine. On each inhale, move the light farther up your spine until it reaches the top of your head. If you ever feel the light fade (your energy level drops), return to the pumping action until your arousal level is up again.
- Once the energy reaches your head, allow it to circle in your brain both clockwise and counterclockwise.
- Touch the tip of your tongue to the roof of your mouth. Stop pumping and experience the flow of energy you have created as it leaves your head and moves down into your solar plexus.

These Eastern sexual traditions may have opened new doors for you and your partner on how to attain and maintain sexual fitness and fulfillment. And there are still more opportunities to experience. In the next chapter, you can learn about the intimate connection between the mind and body and how you can experience sexual health when the two meet.

CHAPTER EIGHT

Mind-Body Sexual Fitness

If you are like most people, when you hear the words "sexual fitness," you envision the physical aspects of sex: making love, the penis and testicles, the vagina and breasts, and whether everything is functioning properly. Although these factors are all important, it ignores the biggest and most important sex organ of all. When that organ is out of sync with the body, chances are your sexual fitness level will be pretty poor. What is that organ? Your mind.

The Mind and Sexual Fitness

The words of Dr. Ruth Westheimer, the world-famous sexologist, are echoed by many of her peers when she says that "The most important sex organ lies between the ears." Most sexual difficulties—approximately 80 percent—are associated with an emotional or psychological cause. When the mind is in turmoil, the body is not far behind.

Fortunately, scientists are discovering more and more about the amazing intimate connection between the body and mind. That knowledge is allowing people to make positive changes in their lives, including their sex lives. Since ancient times, people have known that the mind has the ability to create its own reality, cure the body's ills, or destroy its will to do so. A relatively new branch of science called psychoneuroimmunology studies the relationships among the mind, the nervous system, and the immune system. Researchers have found, for example, that depression can suppress the immune system and make people more susceptible to disease, such as pelvic inflammatory disease, or cause fatigue. Both of these conditions are detrimental to sexual fitness. And there is more.

Performance anxiety for both men and women is an excellent example of how the mind hinders sexual fitness. Most instances of premature ejaculation and lack of sexual desire originate in the mind—emotional issues, problems with stress, anxiety, and tension—and with feeling unable to cope with these problems. Some women do not experience orgasm, not because they are not physically able to do so but because they have been conditioned to believe that "good girls" don't have orgasms or that sex is dirty so they should not enjoy it. Again, the mind can limit sexual fitness.

When people feel they have some control over their lives and the circumstances in them, they are empowered to manage their problems better. Positive thinking, emotions, and attitude promote positive energy and health while their negative counterparts result in fatigue, illness, depression, anger, and fear. Sexual fitness cannot exist in such an environment.

In the rest of this chapter, you will learn about some of the techniques used to link the mind and body for sexual fitness. Qigong, massage, yoga, and sensate focus exercises not only provide a link between body and mind; they infuse a sense of balance and harmony, allowing for the even flow of energy and positive thoughts. Sexual fitness can exist and thrive in such a positive environment. There are many more methods, but the ones presented here are some of the more common ones and the easiest to make a part of your life.

Qigong

If you want to cultivate, control, and make the best use of your sexual energy, learn qigong. This Chinese discipline combines physical training, breathing, visualization, preventive and therapeutic health care, and philosophy into a practice that allows you to maximize your vital essence, or chi.

The word "qigong" means mastery (gong) of the "breath of life" or of the "vital essence" (qi, or chi). Qigong brings together the elements of aerobics, isometrics, isotonics, meditation, and relaxation. The more than 3,000 varieties of qigong fit into five major traditions: Buddhist, Confucian, Taoist, martial arts, and medical. All of the traditions are based on the idea that the human body is an intricate and integrated part of the universe, and qigong's purpose is to maintain that harmonious relationship. The medical tradition is explained here, as it is the most useful for sexual fitness.

Medical qigong combines slow, practiced movements with meditation and breathing exercises. These activities are done together to bring about deep relaxation in which people are aware—but not too aware—of what is happening around them. As tension and stress melt away, positive images, an enhanced spirit, and more self-confidence replace them.

How Qigong Works

Qigong is based on the Chinese philosophy of yin and yang, the opposite yet complementary forces that are part of all nature. When a person's yin and yang are out of balance, the result is dis-ease. Qigong returns the body to balance. Some of the ways it does this is by increasing and improving the flow of oxygen to the body's cells, eliminating muscle tension, reducing stress, and improving organ function. Those who practice qigong learn to build up chi, or vital energy, and send it to areas where their energy is blocked. If this concept sounds familiar, you learned about it in Chapter 7 in the Taoist sex exercises.

As a boost for sexual fitness, qigong normalizes sex hormone levels and can help correct loss of sex drive and impotence. The slow, deliberate movements of qigong help build strength and stamina. Couples who are experiencing stress and anxiety that is having a negative effect on their sex lives can greatly benefit from the stress-relieving powers of qigong.

The practice of qigong also makes people highly sensitive to the internal workings of their body. This heightened sensitivity can be especially helpful for increasing your sexual arousal level.

Qigong for Sexual Vitality

The practice of qigong consists of dozens of movement exercises. You don't need to learn all of the exercises to benefit from qigong, but you do need to practice it, preferably daily. Qigong involves much more than physical training. It requires patience and persistence to integrate your breath and mental processes into the whole healing experience and increase your ability to feel your body, inside and out. The benefits of qigong accumulate over time. Qigong experts say it takes a minimum of three months to appreciate the impact of the exercises.

Before You Start . . .

Practitioners note that because qigong increases blood circulation and thins the blood, women should not practice during menstruation. Others who should not practice qigong include pregnant women, people with acute infectious diseases, or severely mentally disturbed patients. Do not eat or drink at least 90 minutes before a session.

Getting Started

Qigong is a discipline rich in traditions that incorporate the body, mind, and spirit during each session. These traditions are the essence of its effectiveness. Here are some basics to get you started.

- Wear light, comfortable clothing. Shoes are optional; flat shoes with crepe or rubber soles are best.
- Throughout your qigong sessions, face either north or south, which is in line with the earth's magnetic field.
- Exercise at the same time of day and on the same days each week. For the most benefit, practice twice a day for 20 minutes each time. If you have only 5 or 10 minutes, that is preferable to nothing at all.
- Concentrate on your energy center, or solar plexus, throughout each session. In qigong this is referred to as the Dantien. It is the spot just below the belly button and is the storage area for your vital energy.
- Empty your mind of all thoughts and focus only on each motion and your breath. The Chi-

nese believe a quiet mind is essential for qigong to be effective.

- Synchronize your breathing with your movements. This takes practice but becomes very natural once you get used to it. In general, any time you raise your arms or open them up and out, inhale; exhale during any motion that brings your arms close to your body or when you twist your torso.

Qigong for Sexual Fitness

You and your partner can learn dozens of qigong exercises to improve your sexual fitness. Qigong movements are designed to be done in a fluid and graceful sequence, like a ballet. The two representative exercises explained are meant to help you experience the energy and flow of qigong. To get the full impact of this healing art, it is best to take a class or borrow instructional videos you can watch at home.

Flying Wild Goose. This movement strengthens the legs and kidneys, two critical players in sexual fitness.

- Stand straight with your feet hip-width apart, knees slightly bent, and arms comfortably at your sides.
- Raise your arms, elbows, wrists, and then fingers to your sides, up to shoulder level, and breathe in.
- Slowly lower your arms, elbows, wrists, and

then fingers and bend your knees. Breathe out. From this movement you can go naturally into the next.

Rotating the Wheel in a Circle. This movement strengthens the back and makes it more flexible as it moves sexual energy from the solar plexus up the body.

- From the starting position in Flying Wild Goose, bend forward as far as is comfortable, reaching with your fingers toward your toes.
- Slowly bring your arms up and swing them to the left, allowing your right hand to cross in front of your body and your face at about a 45-degree angle. As you raise your arms to the left, rotate your hands so your palms face outward.
- Continue to move your arms in a sweeping motion up over your head and toward the right, allowing your left arm to pass in front of your face and body.
- As your arms reach to the right, begin to bend forward at the waist. Keep your legs straight and don't move your feet. Continue to move slowly down until your hands are pointing straight down to your toes.
- Continue the motion and repeat the circle three to five times in the same direction, then repeat

the entire exercise in the opposite direction an equal number of times.

Massage

Touch is one of the most basic forms of communication among people. It inherently connects people and allows the transfer of energy that can heal, stimulate, and soothe. Massage, especially when shared between sex partners, can be a tremendous boost to sexual fitness and health. The transfer of energy from one partner to another can provide physical, emotional, and spiritual revitalization.

Preparing for Sexual Massage

More than 100 forms of massage exist. The first technique explained here is a slight variation on one from the Taoist tradition. It is designed to awaken the sexual energy of each recipient by stimulating the chakras and moving your sexual energy throughout your body and that of your partner. (Information about other types of massage can be found in the Suggested Readings.) After you and your partner have experienced this massage, your bodies will be in balance and toned for a sexual encounter, if you choose. Allow 30 to 40 minutes for each person to receive the massage.

Before you begin, prepare the massage location: either a massage table or a futon, mattress, or other comfortable arrangement on the floor. You may need several small pillows to prop under your head, knees, or back to maximize your comfort. Also have massage oil on hand. Choose a scent that pleases both of you, or use an unscented general massage oil. Because you will both be nude, make sure the room is warm enough. Create a sensual environment by lighting candles, playing soft music, burning incense, and bringing in flowers.

Massage for Sexual Fitness: For Couples

Note: The instructions are written as if you are the giver.

- Begin with the receiver lying facedown on the floor or massage table. The arms should be lying next to the sides, palms up. Use pillows as needed for comfort.
- You (the giver) begin on the left side of the receiver, kneeling or standing, depending on where the receiver is lying. You will begin by centering yourself and the receiver. To do this, place your left palm in the middle of the receiver's upper back and your right palm on the sacrum (first chakra). While gently massaging both of these areas in a circular motion, synchronize your breathing with that of the receiver. Continue to massage and breathe together for several minutes.

- Apply massage oil to your hands and place both hands, one on top of the other, on the receiver's sacrum (first chakra). Massage the sacrum using small circles and as much pressure as is comfortable for the receiver. Massage in a clockwise or counterclockwise direction. Visualize energy passing from your hands to your partner's body. Ask the receiver to focus on the first chakra and how it feels to receive the energy.
- After several minutes, stop the massage and rest your hands on the receiver's first chakra. Continue to visualize healing energy passing from your hands to your partner. At this point, again synchronize your breathing with that of your partner.
- Apply more oil to your hands and move them up to the second chakra, which is located in the small of the back just below the navel. Repeat the steps you performed at the first chakra: Massage the chakra using circular motion; visualize the energy; stop the massage and rest your hands; synchronize your breathing.
- Repeat this massage sequence for the third chakra (in the small of the back opposite the navel), fourth (middle back opposite the heart), fifth (base of the neck), and sixth (middle back of the head).
- When you reach the seventh chakra (top of the head), gently massage the top of the receiver's

head with your fingertips instead of your palms. Complete the cycle, then switch and become the receiver.

Sexual Massage: Solo

You don't need to have a partner around to enjoy a sexual-fitness massage. Another type of massage that stimulates the flow of vital energy is Oriental massage. The techniques used in Oriental massage unblock areas in the body where energy has become stuck or congested. Once the energy flow is reestablished, sexual energy levels rise, sex organs and hormones function better, and toxins leave the body faster. It can help relieve painful intercourse, impotence, and lack of sexual desire.

The Oriental massage explained next is based on one of two basic approaches. The technique, known as *amma,* involves gentle strokes and rubbing, light pressure, and mild kneading. A more aggressive approach, *tui na,* works at a deeper level. (For more information about Oriental massage, see the Suggested Readings.)

This massage is an abbreviated version of a technique performed by practitioners at the Anhui Medical School in China. Choose a quiet, comfortable location where you can be alone for 10 to 15 minutes. This massage can be done while sitting in a straight-back chair.

SEATED SELF-MASSAGE

- Rub your palms together 30 to 40 times until they are warm.
- Place your warmed palms on your face and, beginning on the left, rub across your forehead to the right side. Repeat this seven or eight times.
- Make a fist with both hands. Place the knuckles of your index and middle fingers of both hands next to the inside of your eyes. Beginning at the inside corner of your eye sockets, use a circular motion to knead around your eye sockets. Move from the inside corner all the way around to the outside corner. Repeat seven to eight times in each direction.
- Place the middle finger of both hands on the indentation on the outside corner of your eyes. Use small circles to knead these two points, making the circles away from and then toward the eyes.
- Place the tips of both middle fingers on the spot from above and between your eyebrows. Make a sweeping motion outward to the points just to the side of your eyes. Repeat this seven or eight times.
- Place the palms of both hands, fingers pointing up, at the hairline on either side of your head, directly above your ears. Press firmly on both sides of your head for one or two seconds, then press on the front and back hairlines. Al-

ternate this pressing motion from the sides to forehead and nape of the neck 30 to 40 times.

- Spread your fingers on both hands and use the flats of your fingers to tap your chest. Inhale each time you tap. Repeat seven to eight times.
- Use the outside edges of both hands to massage your rib cage just below your armpits. Move your hands up and down rapidly in a sawlike motion, doing both sides simultaneously. Go up and down 30 to 40 times.
- Place your left palm over your belly button and place your right hand on the back of the left one. Keeping both hands together, massage your abdomen as deeply as is comfortable in a clockwise direction 30 to 80 times. If you feel any discomfort, discontinue this massage.
- Make fists of both hands, thumbs out, and rapidly chafe both sides of your lower back 30 to 40 times.
- To complete your session, stand with your feet hip-width apart and knees slightly bent. Place your hands in front of you at abdomen height with your palms toward you. Lift your hands toward your throat as you lift your head. Bend backward at the waist and take a deep breath. Hold it for several seconds. Then, as you slowly exhale, lower your hands back to your abdomen, lower your head, and bend forward at the waist. As you exhale, make the sounds

"ha-ho-hee-hoo." Repeat the finishing breath exercise two to four times.

Sensate Focus Exercises

When one or both partners is experiencing a lack of sexual desire, one way to bring the excitement back to the relationship is with sensate focus exercises. These exercises, which are described next, can be done with or without the guidance of a professional sex therapist.

The purpose of the exercises is to help couples focus their minds on each other and the sensations each feels as they explore each other's body. You and your partner should discuss and understand the stages of the exercises before you do them. To be most effective, the stages need to be done as given, and intercourse is banned during the six or more weeks these exercises are practiced.

For all sessions, choose a place and time you will not be disturbed for about 45 minutes. Make the environment as soothing and comfortable as possible; you may want to play soft music, dim the lights, burn aromatic candles, or spritz the room with essential oils. Both you and your partner should be nude during all sessions. Each stage should be practiced at least three times a week for at least two weeks before moving on to the next stage.

Stage 1. The purpose of the initial stage is to learn how to give and receive pleasure. You and your partner can switch off each session as to who will give pleasure and who will receive first.

- While the receiver, or passive partner, lies down comfortably on her stomach, the giver, or active partner, should lubricate his hands with a massage oil or body lotion and kneel next to or astride his partner.
- The giver should begin at the back of the neck and gently massage or stroke his partner's neck, shoulders, back, buttocks, legs, and feet. He can use his hands or tongue. If he does anything that his partner does not like, she should gently push his hand away without speaking. Do the massage and stroking for 10 minutes.
- Now exchange places with your partner—the giver becomes the receiver. Follow the same procedure for 10 minutes.
- Now the couple switches places again, only this time the receiver lies on her back while the giver massages and strokes her body. He should not touch the genitals or breasts. The giver should continue the massage for 10 minutes.
- Once again the partners change places, with the man becoming the receiver. The giver should not touch the genitals during the massage and stroking process. The massage should continue for 10 minutes.

Stage 2. The exchanges of pleasure in this stage are the same as those in stage 1, but this time both partners need to give each other positive feedback about the pleasure they are experiencing. They can do this verbally or by guiding their partner's hand.

- Couples should indicate where they like to be touched and how much pressure they enjoy.
- During this stage partners may kiss, but not on the genitals or female breast.
- At the end of stage 2, partners should discuss what they enjoyed most about the experience.
- Intercourse and touching the genitals are still banned.

Stage 3. By this time, couples should feel very familiar with each other's body as well as their own. During this stage, partners learn to stimulate the genitals.

- While the receiver lies on her back or reclines against her partner's torso, the giver touches and strokes his partner's breasts and genitals. The giver can use his hands and/or mouth to stimulate his partner, but he should not bring his partner to orgasm.
- After 10 minutes the partners switch places and the giver becomes the receiver.

After the couple has practiced stage 3 three times a week for two weeks, they are usually very attuned to each other's sexuality and their own. Now they can move on to intercourse with renewed sexual excitement.

Yoga

More than 5,000 years ago, the ancient Hindus of India developed a mind-body discipline called *yoga*. The literal meaning of the word "yoga" is "union" or "yoking," which signifies the combining of the physical (movement and/or postures) and the emotional/spiritual (breathing and meditation) to reach a higher consciousness.

Types of Yoga

Several different types of yoga exist, yet the most common forms consist of these basic ingredients: stretching movements (called *asanas*), breathing techniques, meditation, and spiritual enlightenment. The practice of yoga simultaneously involves the mind and body, strengthening muscles, improving range of motion, and increasing stamina and flexibility while it calms the mind and fosters internal peace and harmony.

The exercises that follow are from two different traditional forms of yoga. Hatha yoga, which is the most common form in the United States, emphasizes toning and energizing the body using asanas and breathing control. Tantric yoga involves working with the chakras (see Chapter 7) and moving chi, and some

YOGA GUIDELINES

- Practice yoga several times a week. Although one hour is recommended, any time you can spend is worth the effort.
- Wear loose, comfortable clothing and no shoes.
- Wait at least two hours after eating to do yoga.
- Warm up with slow, easy stretches before starting any yoga session.
- Only do what is comfortable. Never force your body into any position.
- Master breath control (see Chapter 7) and be conscious of your breath during your yoga sessions.
- Do yoga on an exercise mat, blanket, or other firm but cushioned flat surface.
- Empty your bladder and bowels before doing yoga.
- To fully appreciate the mind-body connection, always concentrate on your breathing and coordinate it with your movements. It helps to visualize the pose in your mind both before and during the asana.

of the movements focus on sexuality. Tantric yoga exercises are more physical than hatha yoga. They focus on harmonizing the yin and yang—male and female—within each person and between sexual partners. Both hatha and Tantric yoga offer sexual partners opportunities to improve their sexual fitness and response.

Yoga for Sexual Fitness

The Butterfly. This asana makes the hip joints more flexible and tones the inner thighs.

- Sit on the floor and bend your knees. Grasp your feet and draw them toward your pelvis.
- Place the soles of your feet together and allow your knees to fall open.
- Relax your shoulders and keep your back straight.
- Hold this pose and practice the Basic Breath. (See Chapter 7.) Send energy to your pelvis and thighs. With each breath, allow the stretch to increase without causing strain or stress.
- Remain in this pose as long as comfortable, then if you can, go into the Relaxation Pose.

Relaxation Pose. Lie on your back and allow your feet to fall comfortably to each side, about shoulder-width apart. Rest your arms a little away from your sides. If your back is uncomfortable, place a pillow under your knees or bend your knees and bring them together.

- Close your eyes and practice the Basic Breath. Focus on your breath.
- Continue this pose and breath exercise for as long as you desire.

Knee Squeeze. This asana improve circulation to the pelvic region and relaxes the lower back and hips.

- Lie on your back with your arms over your head, resting on the floor.
- Exhale completely and allow your body to sink into the floor.
- Keep your right knee straight as you inhale and bend your left knee. At the same time, lift your head and wrap your arms around the left knee.
- Hold your breath and squeeze your knee to your chest.
- Hold for a count of three, then gently release your knee as you exhale.
- Lower the leg and return your arms to the starting position.
- Repeat the entire sequence with the right knee.
- Do three complete repetitions (three times on each side), then repeat the same exercise lifting both legs at the same time.

Tantric Pelvic Swings. This exercise releases sexual tensions and opens up the pelvic region.

- Kneel on the floor on all fours—with your knees and palms on the floor. Your arms and thighs should be at right angles to the floor. Keep your neck straight; do not let your head hang down.
- Take a slow, deep breath and draw it into your

belly. Tip your head and buttocks up and arch your back. This allows your pelvic area to relax and open.

- Exhale slowly while simultaneously squeezing your buttocks and tipping your pelvis forward and under. This movement causes your back to become rounded and your pelvic muscles to tighten.
- Repeat the cycle 20 or more times: Inhale and open your pelvic region; exhale and squeeze your pelvis.

Tantric Pelvic Swing Two. This is an advanced variation of the last yoga exercise.

- Stand with your legs hip-width apart, knees slightly bent, and your weight evenly distributed.
- Lift your toes, spread them apart, and let them return gently to the floor. Notice how firmly planted you are to the earth.
- Rock back and forth between the balls and heels of your feet. Reaffirm your sense of being grounded.
- Take a breath and send it into your belly. As it enters your belly, swing your pelvis back from your hips. Do not move your legs or waist.
- As you exhale, tighten your abdominal muscles and force out the air in a steady stream. At the

same time, contract your buttocks and tilt your pelvis forward.

- Allow your arms to dangle at your sides. Swing them backward and forward with your pelvis. If this movement is difficult or stiff at first, you will loosen up over time. It may help to practice in front of a mirror so you can focus on swinging your pelvis.
- Practice this exercise every day for 5 to 10 minutes.
- After you have mastered the exercise up to this point, add contraction of your pubococcygeal muscle. When you inhale, open up your pelvic region. As you exhale, squeeze your PC and anal muscles to prevent your sexual energy from leaking out.

EPILOGUE

If you've read this far, you now know that sexual fitness and peak performance are not about whether you came too soon or not at all, or whether you have sex five times a week. It's about sexuality and sensuality that embraces all of your being—physical, mental, emotional, and spiritual. It's about having a deeply satisfying sex life that you and your partner define for yourselves, not what other people tell you it should be. Sexual fitness is a part of everything you do, not just the times you have sex. It is hoped that the remedies, guidelines, and suggestions in this book have shown you how you can enhance your sex life and sexuality in positive, enjoyable, and creative ways.

GLOSSARY

Adrenal Glands. The two small glands situated on top of the kidneys. They produce sex hormones that are responsible for sexual characteristics.

Amino Acids. A group of chemicals that make up the basis of proteins.

Androgens. A term that refers to all of the male sex hormones. In men, the androgens are produced in the testes; in women, a small amount of androgens is produced in the ovaries.

Benign Prostatic Hyperplasia. A noncancerous enlargement of the prostate gland that usually progresses slowly over time.

Bulbourethral Glands. Small glands located below the prostate gland that secrete a clear fluid when men become sexually aroused.

Candidiasis. An infection of the skin or mucus membranes with *Candida*.

Cervix. In the female reproductive system, the term for the neck of the uterus. The cervix separates the uterus from the vagina.

Clitoris. The primary organ for female sexual arousal. This tiny, erectile organ is located below the pubic bone in females.

Corpora Cavernosa. A tissue mass that lies above the corpus spongiosum on both sides of the penile shaft.

Corpus Spongiosum. A tissue mass that lies on the underside of the penis. It is highly sensitive to touch.

Decoction. An herbal remedy prepared from the "tough" parts of the plant, such as the bark, roots, rhizomes, and stems.

Dysmenorrhea. Painful menstrual periods.

Ejaculation. A reflex action that occurs when the penis is stimulated during intercourse or masturbation or spontaneously during sleep and that results in the expulsion of semen.

Epididymis. A collection of tightly coiled tubes, located on top of the testes, which store sperm.

Erection. A process by which the tissues of the penis or clitoris become engorged with blood, causing these organs to become stiff and erect.

Estrogen. A group of hormones found in both men and women that are responsible for sexual development and reproduction. Estrogens (including estradiol, estrone, and estriol) are produced in the adrenal glands in both men and women. They are also made in the ovaries and placenta of women and in the testes of men.

Extract. In herbal medicine and homeopathy, the juice obtained from a plant when it is crushed. Extracts contain a higher concentration of active ingredients than do infusions.

Follicle-Stimulating Hormone. A hormone produced by the pituitary gland of both women and men that causes the gonads to produce ova and sperm.

Glans. The head of the penis.

Gonads. The reproductive organs: the ovaries in women and the testes in men.

G Spot. Theoretically, a highly sexually responsive spot located on the front wall of the vagina between the front of the cervix and the back of the pubic bone.

Impotence. The inability to achieve or maintain an erection. Various psychological and physical problems, as well as drug use, can cause this common male problem.

Infertility. In humans, the inability to conceive after at least 18 months of regular, unprotected sexual intercourse.

Infusion. An herbal remedy, similar to a tea, made from the flowers, leaves, or other soft parts of a plant. Compared with tea, the herbs used in infusions are allowed to steep longer for greater potency.

Labia. The two sets of skin flaps that protect the opening to the vagina. The larger set, labia majora, has pubic hair and sweat glands; the smaller, labia minora, is usually hairless and covers the clitoris.

Libido. Another term for sexual desire.

Masturbation. Sexual self-stimulation practiced by both men and women often to the point of orgasm.

Orgasm. A series of intense physical contractions and sensations that occur at the peak of sexual excitement. In women, the walls of the vagina and uterus contract; in men, the inner pelvic muscles contract.

Penis. The male sex organ through which semen and urine are transported.

Premature Ejaculation. The ejection of semen from the penis either before or soon after the penis achieves penetration.

Progesterone. One of the sex hormones secreted by the ovaries and placenta. It is necessary for the healthy function of a woman's reproductive system.

Prostate Gland. A walnut-size gland located at the neck of the bladder and the urethra in males.

Prostatitis. Inflammation or infection of the prostate gland. The symptoms are similar to those caused by benign prostatic hypertrophy.

Scrotum. A pouch of skin, located behind and under the penis, that contains the testes.

Sexually Transmitted Disease (STD). A disease such as gonorrhea, chlamydia, and AIDS that is transmitted from one person to another through intimate sexual contact.

Testicles (Testes). The two male sex organs that produce sperm and the male sex hormone testosterone. The testicles are located in the scrotum.

Testosterone. A male sex hormone that stimulates sexual development and plays a major role in reproduction. In men it is produced in the testes; in women it is made in much lesser amounts in the ovaries.

Tincture. An extract made with alcohol.

Trans Fatty Acids. Vegetable oils converted into solid fats, also known as partially hydrogenated fats, which are commonly found in margarine and many processed foods.

Uterus. A female reproductive organ that is located behind the bladder and in front of the bowel. It is a hollow, muscular vessel that opens into the vagina at its lower, narrow end and into the fallopian tubes at its upper end. It houses the fetus during pregnancy.

Vagina. The muscular passageway that links the cervix and the external genitalia in the female. It is the structure that the penis enters during intercourse and through which an infant exits during childbirth.

Vaginismus. A type of painful sex that is caused by an involuntary tightening of the vaginal muscles or spastic contractions of the muscles at the vaginal opening.

Vestibular Glands. Tiny glands located on both sides of the vaginal opening that secrete a lubricant when a woman is sexually aroused.

SUGGESTED READINGS

Anand, Margo. *The Art of Sexual Ecstasy*. New York: Tarcher, 1989.

———. *The Art of Sexual Magic*. New York: Tarcher/Putnam, 1995.

Ballentine, Rudolph. *Transition to Vegetarianism: An Evolutionary Step*. Honesdale, Pa.: Himalayan Publishers, 1987.

Barbach, Lonnie. *For Each Other: Sharing Sexual Intimacy*. New York: NAL, 1984.

———. *For Yourself: The Fulfillment of Female Sexuality*. New York: Anchor, 1976.

———. *50 Ways to Please Your Lover While You Please Yourself*. New York: Dutton, 1997.

Balch, James, and Phyllis A. Balch. *Prescription for Nutritional Healing*. Garden City, N.Y.: Avery Publishing, 1990.

Barnard, Neal. *The Power of Your Plate: A Plan for Better Living*. Summertown, Tenn.: Book Publishing, 1995.

Beurdeley, Michel. *The Clouds and the Rain: The Art of Love in China*. London: Hammond, 1969. Published in the United States as *Chinese Erotic Art*. Rutland, Vt.: C. E. Tuttle, 1969.

Chang, Jolan. *The Tao of Love and Sex*. New York: Penguin, 1991.

DePaoli, Carlo. *The Healing Touch of Massage*. New York: Sterling Publishing, 1995.

Dodson, Betty. *Sex for One: The Joy of Selfloving*. New York: Crown, 1996.

Green, James. *Male Herbal*. Freedom, Ca.: The Crossing Press, 1991.

Gulik, R. H. van. *Sexual Life in Ancient China*. Leiden: E. J. Brill, 1961; rev. ed. Atlantic Highlands, N.J.: Humanities Press, 1974.

Harrold, Fiona. *The Complete Body Massage: A Hands-On Manual*. New York: Sterling Publishing, 1992.

Heatherley, Ana Nez. *Healing Plants. A Medicinal Guide to Native North American Plants and Herbs*. New York: Lyons Press, 1998.

Heiman, Julia. *Becoming Orgasmic: A Sexual and Personal Growth Program for Women*. New York: Simon & Schuster, 1988.

Heinerman, John. *Dr. Heinerman's Encyclopedia of Nature's Vitamins & Minerals*. Paramus, N.J.: Prentice-Hall, 1998.

Hewitt, James. *The Complete Yoga Book*. New York: Schocken Books, 1978.

Inkeles, Gordon. *The Art of Sensual Massage*. New York: Simon & Schuster, 1974.

Janus, Samuel S., and Cynthia Janus. *The Janus Report on Sexual Behavior*. New York: John Wiley, 1993.

Lacroix, Nitya. *The Art of Aromatherapy*. New York: Henry Holt, 1995.

Lappe, Frances M. *Diet for a Small Planet*, rev. ed. New York: Ballantine Books, 1975.

Lee, W. E., and Lynn Lee. *Herbal Love Potions: The Magic & Ritual Use of Aphrodisiac Herbs*. Keats Publishing, 1991.

Lockie, Andrew, and Nicola Geddes. *The Women's Guide to Homeopathy*. New York: St. Martin's Press, 1994.

Mayell, Mark. *Natural Energy: A Consumer's Guide to Legal, Mind-Altering, and Mood-Brightening Herbs and Supplements*. New York: Crown Publishers/Random House, 1998.

———. *Off-the-Shelf Natural Health: How to Use Herbs and Nutrients to Stay Well*. New York: Bantam Books, 1995.

McCaleb, Rob. "Herbal Help for Prostate Problems." *Herbs for Health,* Spring/Summer 1996, 26–28.

McIntyre, Anne. *The Complete Woman's Herbal*. New York: Henry Holt, 1994.

Messina, Mark, and Virginia Messina. *The Simple Soybean and Your Health*. Garden City, N.Y.: Avery Publishing, 1994.

Mitchell, Deborah. *Natural Medicine for Diabetes*. New York: Dell, 1997.

Mumford, Jonn. *A Chakra & Kundalini Workbook*. St. Paul, Minn.: Llewellyn Publications, 1994.

Murray, Michael T. *Encyclopedia of Nutritional Supplements*. Rocklin, Ca.: Prima Publishing, 1996.

———. *The Healing Power of Herbs,* 2nd ed. Rocklin, Ca.: Prima Publishing, 1995.

———. *Male Sexual Vitality*. Rocklin, Ca.: Prima Publishing, 1994.

Nefzawi, Shaykh. *The Perfumed Garden*. Translated by Sir Richard Burton. London: Luxor Press, 1963.

Pearsall, Paul. *Sexual Healing*. New York: Crown, 1994.

Prevention editors. *The Female Body: An Owner's Manual*. Emmaus, Pa.: Rodale Press, 1996.

Rako, Susan. *The Hormone of Desire*. New York: Harmony Books, 1996.

Renshaw, Domeena. *Seven Weeks to Better Sex*. New York: Random House, 1995.

Robbins, John. *Diet for a New America: How Your Food Choices Affect Your Health, Happiness, and the Future of Life on Earth*. Walpole, N.H.: Stillpoint Publishing, 1987.

———. *May All Be Fed*. New York: Morrow, 1992; Avon, 1993.

Sachs, Judith. *The Healing Power of Sex*. Englewood Cliffs, N.J.: Prentice-Hall, 1994.

Shealy, C. Norman. *The Illustrated Encyclopedia of Healing Remedies*. Boston: Element Books, 1998.

Stoppard, Miriam. *The Magic of Sex*. New York: Dorling Kindersley, 1992.

Swift, Rachel. *How to Have an Orgasm . . . as Often as You Want*. Carroll & Graf, 1993.

Tappan, Frances. *Healing Massage Techniques*. Norwalk, Conn.: Appleton & Lange, 1988.

Tierra, Lesley. *The Herbs of Life: Health and Healing Using Western and Chinese Techniques*. Freedom, Ca.: The Crossing Press, 1992.

———. *The Way of Herbs*. New York: Simon & Schuster, 1990.

Tisserand, Maggie. *Essence of Love: Fragrance, Aphrodisiacs, and Aromatherapy for Lovers*. San Francisco: Harper, 1994.

Walker, Richard. *The Family Guide to Sex and Relationships*. New York: Macmillan, 1996.

Watson, Cynthia Mervis. *Love Potions: A Guide to Aphrodisiacs and Sexual Pleasures,* New York: Jeremy Tarcher/Perigree, 1993.

Werbach, Melvyn. *Healing Through Nutrition*. New York: HarperCollins, 1993.

———. *Nutritional Influences on Illness,* 2nd ed. Tarzana, Ca.: Third Line Press, 1993.

Whitaker, Julian. *Dr. Whitaker's Guide to Natural Healing*. Rocklin Ca.: Prima Publishing, 1995.

Wildwood, Christine. *Flower Remedies: Natural Healing with Flower Essences*. Boston: Element Books, 1991.

Yaffe, Maurice, and Elizabeth Fenwick. *Sexual Happiness for Men*. New York: Henry Holt, 1992.

———. *Sexual Happiness for Women*. New York: Henry Holt, 1992.

APPENDIX A

Organizations and Other Sources of Information

EASTERN SEXUAL TRADITIONS

SkyDancing Institute
20 Sunnyside Avenue, Suite A219
Mill Valley, CA 94941
415–927–2584; or 800–927–2584
Tantric seminars and training programs; ritual accessories

FOOD, FOOD SAFETY, AND SUPPLEMENTS

American Academy of Orthomolecular Medicine
900 North Federal Highway
Boca Raton, FL 33432
800–847–3802

American Natural Hygiene Society
PO Box 30630
Tampa, FL 33630
813–855–6607

Center for Science in the Public Interest
1875 Connecticut Avenue NW, Suite 300
Washington, DC 20009
202–332–9111
Publishers of *The Nutrition Action Health Letter*

"Food, Nutrition, and the Prevention of Cancer: A Global Perspective." For a free brochure about the report, call the American Institute for Cancer Research, 800–843–8114, ext. 121, and ask for the food nutrition study publication.

National Coalition Against the Misuse of Pesticides
701 E. Street SE, Suite 200
Washington, DC 20003
202–543–5450
Information on the health effects and alternatives to pesticides.

National Coalition for Alternatives to Pesticides
PO Box 1393
Eugene, OR 97440
503–344–5044
Information on nontoxic ways to eliminate hazards introduced by fungi and pests.

Natural Food Associates
PO Box 210
Atlanta, TX 75551
800–594–2136

North American Vegetarian Society
PO Box 72
Dolgeville, NY 13329
518–568–7970

Physicians Committee for Responsible Medicine
PO Box 6322
Washington, DC 20015
202–686–2210

Preventive Medicine Research Institute
Dean Ornish, MD
900 Bridgeway, Suite 2
Sausalito, CA 94965
415–332–2525

Soy Protein Council
1255 23rd Street NW, Suite 850
Washington, DC 20037
202–467–6610

United Soybean Hotline
800–TALK–SOY
Recipes and information about soy and soy products

Vegetarian Education Network
PO Box 3347
West Chester, PA 19380
215–696–VNET

Vegetarian Resource Group
PO Box 1463
Baltimore, MD 21203
410–366–8343

HERBS AND HOMEOPATHY

American Botanical Council
PO Box 201660
Austin, TX 78720
800–373–7105

Organizations and Other Sources of Information

American Foundation for Homeopathy
1508 Glencoe Street, Suite 44
Denver, CO 80220–1338

American Herb Association
PO Box 1673
Nevada City, CA 95959
916–265–9552

American Herbalists Guild
PO Box 1683
Soquel, CA 95073
408–464–2441

Herb Research Foundation
1007 Pearl Street, Suite 200
Boulder, CO 80302
303–449–2265

Homeopathic Academy of Naturopathic Physicians
14653 South Graves Road
Mulino, OR 97042
503–829–7326

Homeopathic Educational Services
2124 Kittredge Street
Berkeley, CA 94704
800–359–9051

National Center for Homeopathy
801 N. Fairfax Street, Suite 306
Alexandria, VA 22314
703–548–7790

MIND-BODY

American Massage Therapy Association
1130 West North Shore Avenue
Chicago, IL 60626
312–761–AMTA

American Oriental Bodywork Association
6801 Jericho Turnpike
Syosset, NY 11791
516–364–5533

Associated Bodywork & Massage Professionals
28677 Buffalo Park Road
Evergreen, CO 80439
800–458–2267

Himalayan Institute of Yoga, Science and Philosophy
RR1 Box 400
Honesdale, PA 18431
717–253–5551
Catalog; also publishes the magazine *Yoga International*

International Association of Yoga Therapists
109 Hillside Avenue
Mill Valley, CA 94941
415–383–4587

SEX AND SEXUALITY

American Association for Marriage and Family Therapy
1133 15th Street, Suite 300
Washington, DC 20005
202–452–0109
Web site: http://www.aamft.org
Offer referrals to therapists or clinics

Organizations and Other Sources of Information

American Association of Sex Educators, Counselors and Therapists
PO Box 238
Mount Vernon, IA 52314
319–895–8407
Web site: http://www.aasect.org
Offers referrals to therapists or clinics

Kinsey Institute for Research in Sex, Gender, and Reproduction
Indiana University
Morrison Hall, Third Floor
Bloomington, IN 47405
812–855–7686
Web site: http://www.indiana.edu/~kinsey/
Offers information on sexuality

Phoenix Counsel
Linda Crabtree
1 Springback Drive
St. Catharines, Ontario, Canada L2S 2K1
It's Okay! a magazine on sexuality and disability

Sexuality Information and Education Council of the U.S.
130 West 42nd Street, Suite 2500
New York, NY 10036
212–819–9770
Web site: http://www.siecus.org
Offers information on sexuality

APPENDIX B

Product Sources

HERBAL AND HOMEOPATHIC SOURCES

Frontier Cooperative Herbs
3021 78th Street
PO Box 299
Norway, IA 52318
800–669–3275
Web site: http://www.natnet.com/fronteit/

Gaia Herbs
12 Lancaster Country Road
Harvard, MA 01451
800–831–7780

The Herb Pharm
PO Box 116
Williams, OR 97544
800–348–4372

Herbs, Etc.
1345 Cerrillos Road
Santa Fe, NM 87505
888–694–3727

San Francisco Herb Company
250 14th Street
San Francisco, CA 94103
800–227–4530

ORGANIC AND PLANT-BASED FOOD PRODUCERS

Arrowhead Mills
PO Box 2059
Hereford, TX 79045
806–364–0730
Organic grains and flours

Eden Foods
701 Tecumseh Road
Clinton, MI 492236
517–456–7424

ORGANIC FOODS; SOY-BASED FOODS, SOY BEVERAGES

Ivy Foods
7613 South Prospector Drive
Salt Lake City, UT 84121
801–943–7664
Wheat-based "meat" products

Morningstar Farms
Worthington Foods
Worthington, OH 43085
614–885–9511

MEATLESS PRODUCTS: BREAKFAST LINKS, BREAKFAST PATTIES, DELI FRANKS, AND OTHERS

Nasoya
800–229–8638
Tofu, Nayonaisse

Purity Foods
2871 W. Jolly Road
Okemos, MI 48864
800–99–SPELT
Pastas

Soyco Foods
2441 Viscount Row
Orlando, FL 32809
407–855–6600
Cheese alternatives

Westbrae (soy beverages)
800–769–6455

White Wave
1990 N. 57th Court
Boulder, CO 80301
303–443–3470
Meatless chicken products

INDEX

ABOUT THE AUTHOR

DEBORAH MITCHELL is a writer and editor whose medical and health-related articles have appeared in consumer and professional journals. She was the ghostwriter for *The Good Sex Book*, and author of other books, including *The Natural Health Guide to Headache Relief*, *Natural Medicine for PMS*, *Natural Medicine for Weight Loss*, *Natural Medicine for Back Pain*, and *Nature's Aphrodisiacs*. She lives in Tucson, Arizona.

ALSO AVAILABLE

BOOST YOUR SEXUAL ENERGY

by Judith Sachs

ISBN: 0-7434-9769-4

Did you know that sex can dramatically boost your overall well-being? If you, like many people, are hitting midlife and feeling that sex is just not what it used to be, think again. While you are experiencing a variety of physical and emotional changes, sex can still be one of the enduring pleasures you can enjoy through midlife and on to your golden years.

This unique guide provides important information on age-related changes in sexual function and offers a wide range of medical, holistic, and psychological tips and techniques that can relight your fire. Don't miss:

- Testosterone cream that restores a woman's libido
- Zinc, the most important mineral for male potency, and all the must-have nutrients
- The best herbal alternatives to Viagra™
- Ways to fulfill sexual needs if there is illness or disability
- The Seesaw and other stimulating exercises to make sex feel great